Life's Journey

Kathy Herzog

iUniverse, Inc.
Bloomington

Life's Journey

iUniverse books may be ordered through booksellers or by contacting:

iUniverse
1663 Liberty Drive
Bloomington, IN 47403
www.iuniverse.com
1-800-Authors (1-800-288-4677)

ISBN: 978-1-4620-7288-0 (sc)
ISBN: 978-1-4620-7286-6 (hc)
ISBN: 978-1-4620-7287-3 (e)

Printed in the United States of America

iUniverse rev. date: 1/6/2012

Contents

Chapter 1

New Beginnings

The story of my life is not so different from many other women's lives. However, not many women could say they have been married three times and became a widow at thirty-five. This is my story. I hope that by sharing my narrative, other women in similar situations will find comfort and strength when it seems there isn't any to be found.

Raised in a small town in north central Wisconsin, I was naive and not aware of what happens when a young woman is out on her own for the first time.

Yes, I had gone to college for two years prior to moving to Illinois. In college, I experienced beer parties and dorm life, but I had no idea what it was like to be in a serious relationship. I was accustomed to being independent and not having to answer to anyone about my whereabouts. I enjoyed this freedom and was not ready to face the journey ahead of me.

In January 1990, I began working as a live-in nanny for a couple who had three children. I enjoyed caring for their three-year-old daughter and twins who were six weeks old when I started my employment. The freedom of living on my own and being responsible enough to be entrusted with the care of children felt terrific. I enjoyed having my weekends off, and I began to explore the social activities that the small town in northern Illinois offered.

At first, it was difficult to get to know people. How does a single young woman go about meeting people and making friends? I decided to attend one of the local clubs in town and see what the atmosphere was like. The loud music and various people were exciting to me. I enjoyed watching others dance and would sit at the bar and slowly sip a beer or wine cooler while listening to the beat of the music.

After hanging out at this club for several months, a very tall, thin, balding guy approached me. He asked if I would like to dance, and I excitedly accepted his invitation. We danced to a couple of fast songs and then made our way back to the bar.

We started a casual conversation about where we worked and what our hobbies were. It was nice to meet someone new, and we enjoyed each other's company. At the end of the evening, Jim asked for my phone number, and I gave it to him without a second thought.

It was early the next week when Jim called to see if I would like to go out with him. I accepted his invitation, and we met the following weekend at his house. It was small and clean, and I had the impression that he had cleaned just to impress me. We actually stayed in and watched a movie on television. The night was casual, and at the end of our date, Jim kissed me. I was surprised and a little taken aback. Was this normal? Were things moving a little too fast? I had nothing to compare this relationship to, so I just went with the flow.

Jim and I began dating on a regular basis. Sometimes we would go out to the local club. Other times we would meet at his house. There was more privacy at his place than trying to find privacy at the home where I was working as a nanny.

One Saturday afternoon, Jim and I went to Rockford, Illinois, to look at vintage records. Jim had a record collection and wanted me to share the experience of looking for records with him. It must have been pretty evident that I was bored with the entire shopping escapade, because I heard him whisper to the clerk, "I don't think she would be here if she weren't here with me." This was true. I hadn't ever pictured myself in a record store looking at albums that were older than I was.

My relationship with Jim continued on a steady basis. Typically, we would see each other only on weekends, because we were both busy with our jobs during the week.

One evening as we were sitting at his home, the mood became very sensual. Jim and I began making out and kissing a lot. The next thing I knew, he was asking me if I wanted to go to the bedroom and have intercourse. Not the romantic way I had envisioned getting to know a guy. Honestly, we had been intimate before, but I was having my period at the time and had no interest in any sexual encounters that evening. Then Jim said, "Well, how about if you just please me in other ways?"

I was horrified and disappointed. Never before had I experienced this, and I really didn't know what to do. The first thought that came to my head was, *Get the hell out of here.* So I made up some lame excuse about being tired and left.

Shortly after that date, my feelings for Jim changed. I no longer felt comfortable around him. So one evening when he called me on the telephone, I told him that I didn't want to see him anymore. He reluctantly accepted my feelings, and we said our good-byes after a very brief conversation.

Even though this relationship did not work out, at the ripe age of twenty-two, I believed I really knew what I wanted out of life. I had a job I loved and felt like I was on top of the world.

Chapter 2

Dating Experiences

During the summer of 1990, I met a thin, lonely guy at one of the clubs in a small town in southern Wisconsin. I was tired of hanging out at the local club and wanted to get some different socializing experiences. As I hung out at the bar nursing a wine cooler, I stared off into space and listened to music selected by the disc jockey. I admit, I must have looked lonely and out of my element. I wasn't a regular at this club, and I tried to look like I was having a good time. In reality, I was bored and regretted my decision to come to the club in the first place.

However, after a short while, Mark came up and asked if I would like to dance. This guy was not my type, but he seemed just as bored and lonely as I was, so I accepted his invitation. After dancing to a few songs, Mark asked if he could buy me a drink. I accepted, and we started talking about our jobs and other various subjects. It was getting late, and I was ready to head home. I had at least a thirty-minute drive, and I was tired. Mark asked me for my phone number, and I gave it to him thinking that he most likely wouldn't call me.

The next day he called and asked if I would like to meet him at his house. I was pleasantly surprised and a little apprehensive as well. Sure, we had talked the night before, and I had found out that Mark was legally separated from his wife. He also had a daughter who was two years old. I didn't have a problem with him having a child, but in the back of my mind, I kept second-guessing my decision to go on a date with him. This guy was still legally married to someone else. This little voice told me, *Kathy, he's still married; maybe you should wait until he is divorced to date him.*

However, I ignored that little voice and accepted Mark's invitation to visit him at his house. I arrived a little after 7:00 p.m. Mark was playing with his daughter and getting her settled in for the night. What struck me was how calm and devoted he was to his daughter. He seemed to be a very caring and happy father despite the problems he was having with his wife.

Mark and I played with his daughter for a little while longer, and then he put her to bed. I waited patiently while he tucked her in and got her settled for the night. The television was on, so I sat on the couch, watching the show on the screen.

When Mark came from the bedroom, he apologized for the wait. I told him it was no problem. I knew that children were a first priority, and making time for a spouse or girlfriend, whatever the case may be, is second. Mark and I cuddled on the couch, and he told me more about his recent separation. He and his wife couldn't make it work but were still legally married until they could pay off some debts. This was understandable. However, I still felt guilty about dating someone who was still legally married.

Again, I pushed those thoughts aside because I really liked Mark and wanted to get to know him better.

Mark and I started dating on a regular basis. Sometimes I would travel to southern Wisconsin to see him, and other times he would drive to the town where I was living in northern Illinois. It was becoming a comfortable relationship, and we both enjoyed spending time with each other.

For my birthday in July, Mark took me to a fancy Italian restaurant in the town I lived. The restaurant was quite expensive, and I commented on how good the food was. Mark said, "Well, I hope so, because this cost me a lot." This remark made me feel guilty, because I knew he was already stretched beyond his financial means. But he could have recommended a less expensive place for dinner, and I would have been just as happy.

The week after my birthday, I traveled back to my hometown in north central Wisconsin. I enjoyed the time visiting friends and family. My parents and I talked about my relationship with Mark. I told them that he was not yet divorced but was legally separated from his wife. I also told them that he had a young daughter. My parents didn't tell me not to go out with Mark anymore; they said it was my decision but that I should think seriously about this relationship. *Did I want to be a stepmother if this relationship was serious? Would I be happy dating this guy until he got a divorce?*

These thoughts weighed heavily on my mind as I drove back to northern Illinois after my weeklong vacation. I kept thinking about what my parents had said. *Did I really feel good about this relationship?* Truthfully, the answer was no. I kept convincing myself on the drive back to Illinois that I needed to break up with Mark as soon as possible.

Once I arrived in Illinois and unpacked, I decided to call Mark. I couldn't put off the inevitable. I'd feel better about the whole situation if I went through with the breakup and moved on. I dialed Mark's number. I was nervous and apprehensive and thought, *Will I sincerely be able to tell him how I feel?* Mark answered the phone and asked me about my vacation. I told him it was fine.

Hesitantly, I told Mark that I didn't think we should see each other any more. He paused a few seconds, and then he said, "I think you have had other people influencing your decision—am I right?"

I tried to deny that remark and told him that, no, this was my decision. Mark asked if he could come see me and talk about this. Standing firm in my conviction, I told him that a discussion wouldn't be a good idea. Mark was clearly disappointed and eager to see me again. Finally, I convinced him that our relationship was over.

Chapter 3

Back on the Dating Wagon

For the next few months, I took a break from dating. I needed to clear my mind and think about my priorities. My job as a nanny meant a lot to me, and I wanted to be a responsible, caring caregiver to the children. But I also wanted to socialize and meet people in the community. I did talk with one of my employer's friends and we got along very well, but she was married and expecting her first child, so we didn't have much in common.

At the end of August, I decided to go back to the local club in town and see what was going on. I remember it was an extremely sticky, hot summer evening and I dressed to impress. I wore a short denim skirt and blouse. The ensemble looked nice, but was not comfortable for a hot evening. However, I was enjoying myself at the bar, nursing a wine cooler, and listening to the dance music.

After a little while, a tall, thin guy with curly, long brown hair came up and asked me if I wanted to dance. I accepted his invitation, and we danced to several fast songs. Alex and I made our way back to the bar, and he said, "Darlin', would you like another drink?" His southern drawl was sexy. We both got another drink and continued making small talk at the bar. Alex lit a cigarette and continued his conversation with ease. It was very easy and fun to talk with this guy. He was charming and very attentive to our conversation.

Alex and I talked some more, and then we went out on the dance floor a few more times. He asked for my phone number, and I gave it to him at the end of the evening without another thought.

Early the next week, Alex called and asked if we could go on a date. He had purchased tickets for Great America and wanted me to go along with him. "Sure," I said. "That sounds like fun!"

Alex told me that we could leave from his apartment on Saturday at around 9:00 a.m. That entire week I was giddy and excited. I had just met this guy who treated me like a princess. *Was this too good to be true?*

On Friday evening after work, I met Alex at his apartment. I had my bag of clothes packed and was ready for a fun weekend. That evening we went out for dinner. It was nothing fancy, but we talked and had a good time. We arrived back at Alex's apartment and he offered me one of his oversize T-shirts to wear to bed. I didn't know what to think; were we moving too fast? However, my fears quickly dissolved when Alex and I went to bed and slept the entire night.

The next morning we were both up bright and early. I was super excited, and Alex was in a good mood too. He didn't have a vehicle, so he drove my car since he knew where we were going. This was fine with me, because my sense of direction is terrible and I would have gotten us lost in no time.

On our drive, we talked about various things. Alex talked about his children. Yes, he had twins who were twenty-two, about the same age as I was. This surprised me, but I didn't really see a problem with it since I didn't think I would ever become a stepmother to his children. In fact, Alex hadn't seen his kids since they were about eight years old. He and his ex-wife had divorced, and there were some ill feelings between them. This also meant that there was about a twenty-year age difference between Alex and myself. This didn't bother me either, as I consider age to be irrelevant. You can feel and act like you're sixty even when you're forty if you don't take care of yourself and eat right. Alex was very fit and had a very active lifestyle.

Alex asked me if I had ever been to Great America. The last time I had been there was when I was in grade school, which had been many years ago.

Once we got to our destination, Alex parked my car in one of the parking lots near the amusement park. I was amazed at the big roller coasters. You could see them from the highway.

Alex paid for our tickets, and we headed off for a day of fun and excitement. I am not a big fan of carnival rides or roller coasters. But I felt protected and secure with Alex beside me holding my hand. We enjoyed walking around the amusement park and going on many of the rides. Alex bought us lunch, and we enjoyed talking and getting to know each other even more.

By the end of our day together, I was infatuated with Alex's suave southern charm. He had called me darlin' on several occasions, and this endearment made me feel very special. As Alex drove home that evening, we talked some more, and I felt happier than I had in a long time.

Alex and I spent the remaining weekend together. His bachelor pad left a lot to be desired. I was used to having a lot of room to myself. His apartment was no bigger than the entire basement of the house I was living in during this time! The apartment had one bedroom, a small living room, and a bath with no shower. It also had a certain flashback vibe to the seventies, a shag rug and brown furniture scattered throughout the apartment.

Our relationship continued to grow throughout the month of September. I would take the little girl I was caring for to preschool, and then visit Alex before I returned home to attend to other household duties. Each weekend, Alex and I would spend the entire time together at his apartment.

Alex soon came up with a nickname for me. He began to call me Katie, and it stuck like glue. Each time he introduced me to someone new, I was his girlfriend Katie. But this bothered my parents, because at the time we had a dog named Katie. My parents questioned why Alex had to use this nickname. I tried to assure them that it was just a nickname and not a big deal.

During the first few weeks of October 1990, the family I was working for decided to move to Minnesota. They had a home there, and the wife had just gotten a promotion, which required the family to move back to their hometown. I was disappointed and excited at the same time. I didn't want to leave Alex and move so far away. Our relationship was still growing, and I didn't want to be away from him for too long. However, I had an employment contract and needed to fulfill my duties at least until December of that year.

Chapter 4

Marriage Proposal

One morning in early October, when I went to visit Alex at his apartment, he took out a small ring box. Inside was a beautiful, antique-looking wedding ring. Alex said, "Katie, will you marry me?"

I was shocked and a little apprehensive. We hadn't been dating that long, but I quickly accepted Alex's proposal. He placed the ring on my finger and gave me a long, tender kiss. I stared in disbelief at the diamond on my finger. *Was this real? Was I making a solid decision?* I knew that in a couple of weeks I would be moving to Minnesota with the family who employed me. At the time, this was my reassurance that Alex would be in Illinois waiting for me when my contract was up in December.

During dinner with the family the next evening, I mentioned my engagement and upcoming plans to my employers. Bryce, the dad, looked at me with fatherly concern and said, "I don't think this is a good idea; you really don't know this guy that well."

His wife looked at him and then at me and said, "Bryce, this is Kathy's decision, and if this is what she wants to do, then we don't have anything to say about it."

I also told them that at the end of December, I would be moving back to Illinois, because my contract as a nanny was up. They both understood my position, but I could tell Bryce still wasn't sure this was the best decision for me.

I was in love and that was all that mattered. Alex's southern charm had won me over. I was engaged and I planned to get married. For the next several weeks, I spent as much free time as I could with Alex. I also packed up my belongings for the anticipated move to Excelsior, Minnesota, at the end of October.

The evening before our move to Minnesota, I went to Alex's apartment to tell him good-bye. I sat in his arms and cried my eyes out. I kept telling him, "I'll miss you so much. I don't want to leave you."

Alex cuddled me in his arms and said, "It's only a couple months, and then we'll be together again."

I wasn't too sure about this whole move to Minnesota. I felt so connected to Alex, and I didn't want to spend any time away from him.

Chapter 5

Moving Again

The next day, the moving van arrived to gather the family's belongings. I followed in my car. The trip took six hours, but we stopped several times to eat and to make sure the kids were changed and comfortable. We arrived at the house in Minnesota early that evening. I was amazed at how big the house was! It was a huge white house with so many windows I was unable to count them all. I helped get the children settled and then went downstairs to scope out my bedroom. Just like at the other house, I had my own living area. It was very comfortable and offered plenty of room for me. I liked the big bed, and I had a bathroom to myself.

During that first weekend in our new home, I unpacked my room and started getting familiar with the layout of the house. The twins shared a big bedroom upstairs. The little girl had her own bedroom that began to take on a very girly feel. The children adjusted very well to their new surroundings. I had to keep a close eye on the toddling twins, as there were so many more stairs and obstacles for them to overcome.

I wasn't prepared for the cold, wintery weather that invades Minnesota. We got quite a bit of snow and cold weather during the first few weeks of November. I would venture out on weekends and check out the mall. I also tried to keep fit by exercising on the stair-stepper in my room. I was lonely and bored. Alex wrote me long letters each week telling me how much he missed me and telling me what was happening at home. I would write him back faithfully, telling him that I missed him a lot too.

At the beginning of December, the family and I worked together to hire a different nanny. She would officially begin her duties in mid-December, and then I would leave and move back to Illinois.

I taught the new nanny the routine I had with the children. In the mornings, I would take the little girl to preschool. When I returned, I would help give the twins a bath. Then I would work on doing laundry before going to pick up Chelsea from preschool again. Next, we would eat lunch, and then I would put the twins and Chelsea down for an afternoon nap. In the afternoon, I would fold laundry, prepare supper, and play with the children before their parents returned home from work.

Sometimes I left the household chores undone while I cared for a tired, hungry, or fussy child. I enjoyed my job, and I tried to encourage the new nanny the importance of making sure that the children always came first.

Chapter 6

Life with Alex

By the second week of December, my time with the Bradford family was finished. I said my good-byes to the parents before they left for work. In the early afternoon, I helped settle the children down for their afternoon nap and said my good-byes to them as well. Leaving a family I had grown to care for during the past year was very emotional. But at the same time, I was excited to start my life with Alex in Illinois. I drove most of the afternoon and early evening before finally arriving at Alex's apartment.

Alex and I were so happy to see each other after our time apart. I was happy to be with him again, and a small part of me didn't want Alex to go to work that evening. I wanted to spend as much time with him as possible. However, I knew I was being selfish and finally allowed Alex to go to work.

I settled into my life with Alex pretty well. While he slept during the day, I checked out returning to college for the spring semester. There was a four-year college in Rockford, Illinois. It was about a thirty-minute drive from where we were living. I could take classes during the day and work a part-time job to help pay for the bills and groceries. I hadn't realized just how expensive it was to return to college. It would cost approximately $11,000 to attend college for the spring semester! I hoped I would get some financial aid to help pay for tuition.

My relationship with Alex continued to grow throughout the winter months. I started taking classes at Rockford College in mid-January 1992. The drive wasn't too bad, but a few days the winter weather made driving somewhat dicey. I also started working part-time at a daycare center in

Rockford. As part of my work-study and financial aid package, I also worked in the administration office helping with paperwork and answering the telephone when my boss was out of the office.

I really enjoyed my classes, especially Classroom Management. I learned techniques that would help me once I got into a classroom setting and began to teach students. Alex was not supportive of me going back to college. I was spending a lot of time studying and working and not spending as much time with him.

I could tell that Alex was building up some resentment toward me. He had never had the opportunity to finish college and seeing me pursue my education pissed him off. Alex only saw how much money and effort I was putting into my education. He didn't understand that furthering my education would benefit us in the long run. Later on, I would get a teaching job that would provide us with more money and a secure future.

Chapter 7

The Breakup

During spring break, I went home to visit my parents. They could tell I was upset and a little disappointed in Alex. I decided that I would break up with Alex and continue the rest of the semester at college living in a dorm room. When I broke it off with Alex in late March, he was very upset with me. He didn't understand why education was so important to me. In fact, I told him I wanted to finish my degree. He replied by telling me that he wanted to win the lottery. Maybe he thought that my getting an education was as unattainable as winning the lottery. I'm not sure how the two relate. But I plugged away at my studies feeling lonely and unsure about my decision to break up with Alex.

One weekend in mid-April, I decided to go to Alex's apartment and get some of my stuff. He was home and we started talking. One thing led to another and before I knew what was happening we were back together again. I continued attending classes at Rockford College, but neglected to tell my parents that Alex and I were back living together again. My parents had helped pay for my college tuition and were livid when I told them that I had moved back to Alex's apartment. I had literally wasted a lot of the money they were contributing to my education.

Chapter 8

Getting Married

Alex and I decided to get married at the end of May 1992. Since my family had taken such a dislike to him, I decided not to tell them or invite them to the wedding. The ceremony was a very small affair held at the city park on May 29, 1992. We were married by an African American Baptist minister with two of Alex's friends as our witnesses.

I wore a simple, long-sleeved white dress that I had bought at Fashion Bug. Alex bought and wore a sage green suit for the service. After the ceremony, we went home and changed clothes, and then Alex took me to one of the local bars for dinner and dancing. That evening as we were dancing, Alex excused himself to use the bathroom. I began to get concerned when he didn't come back for quite some time. When Alex returned, I thought he was acting a little weird, flighty, and high. He admitted that he had just smoked pot in the bathroom with a buddy of his. I was hurt and a little disappointed. This was our wedding night, and Alex had gone off and gotten high while I sat around waiting for him.

During that summer, I continued to work at a daycare center in Rockford. However, as the summer ended, Alex and I discussed me going back to college. There was no way we could afford the tuition at Rockford College, so I decided that I would take a few classes at the community college in our hometown and find a part-time job to help make ends meet.

Fortunately, I found a job working in an after school daycare program. This arrangement fit well with my schedule. I took classes in the morning and early afternoon, and then worked at the daycare center from three to six. Alex still resented the fact that I wanted to continue with my education. He felt I was spending too much time working and studying and not enough time with him! We got into a fight one afternoon just before I went off to class. Alex asked, "Why is it so important for you to go to school?"

I tried to explain that this would benefit our future, and I would get a better job once I earned my degree. But Alex didn't want to hear that and called me a spoiled rotten child.

Chapter 9

Relationship Problems

Yes, it is true my parents had always provided everything for me, but now I was married and had responsibilities. I knew Alex cared about me, but I slowly came to realize that we wanted different things from life. For the next two years, I worked at a daycare center and left my college plans behind. It was more important to me to make Alex happy and help provide income for our financial needs.

However, as time passed, I began to resent the fact that I couldn't do what I wanted with my life. I also disliked Alex's excessive drinking and partying. One evening we were invited to a house party. I didn't really know any of the people at the party except the host. Alex and his friend had been playing pool, but somehow I lost track of Alex. He came back by me a while later with a glazed stare. I knew this look, the look of a pot smoker, someone who was high. Alex stared at me and said, "Once a pothead, always a pothead." This was supposed to make me feel better and excuse his behavior. Once again, I felt like I was second fiddle to his partying lifestyle.

Alex and I also discussed trying to have children, but each time I broached the subject, it was pushed to the back burner. He had two children from his previous marriage and didn't seem too anxious to start another one. Once when I asked him about having kids he said, "I like things how they are. Why can't you just be happy with the way it is?"

There were several instances where Alex and I had some terrible verbal fights. I would call him an a**hole, and he would call me a spoiled brat. During our almost five years of marriage, I became frighteningly aware that the man I married was someone very different from the husband I had. Alex was an alcoholic, a drug abuser, and had become verbally abusive to me over the years.

One weekend at my parents' house, I sat down at the kitchen table and had a good cry. After many tears and several hours of soul-searching, I decided to leave my husband, move back to my hometown, and start a new chapter in my life. The only request I had of my parents was that they not tell me "we told you so." Both of my parents had never really liked Alex and had tried to discourage me from marrying him in the first place. But I was young, had been in love, and that was all that mattered to me at the time.

Chapter 10

Starting Over

I moved back to my hometown in March 1996. I wanted desperately to give myself a fresh start. I remember the first month as being difficult. I couldn't find a job, and I was getting very restless being around my parents all the time. Then at the end of April, I found a job at one of the local factories. I vowed that I would save up enough money to go back to school in January 1997.

During the next several months, I worked hard and learned to appreciate the things I had. Factory work wasn't something I wanted to do the rest of my life. I knew that I needed to return to college to obtain my bachelor's degree.

In the winter of 1996, I frequented a few of the local bars and one night a guy introduced himself to me. Why I decided to date him I will never really understand. Once again, I was lonely and wanted to share some time with someone who cared about me. We dated for almost two months before I returned to college.

The winter of 1997 was both a strange and exciting time for me. For the first time, I felt independent and free to choose what I wanted to do with my life. When I went through with my divorce, I picked up the nasty habit of smoking. So I spent many hours in my dorm room smoking and learning what I needed to do to get the degree that I wanted. I attended classes four days a week and worked part-time at one of the daycare centers in Sheboygan. For the first time in many years, I felt good about myself.

Chapter 11

Dating Once Again

My divorce was finalized in April 1997, and I continued to date the guy who I had met at the bar in November of the previous year. I tried really hard to make this relationship work, but the physical distance between us and his excessive drinking and drug use only made me feel used once again. So in June we broke up. I felt I was leading myself down another path toward self-destruction, and I didn't want to make the same mistakes all over again.

During that summer, I met a guy and we hit it off instantly. The first night we met, we spent hours talking at the bar until closing time! Kin called me up the next day and asked me on a date. That summer was very exciting for me. For the first time, I was dating a guy who truly liked me and didn't have drug or alcohol problems. Kin was very spontaneous and took me on road trips to various parts of Wisconsin. I didn't mind too much, but I am the kind of person who likes things to be planned out. So it took me a while to get used to Kin's spontaneous behavior.

The fall of 1997 quickly approached, and I knew I would be going back to college soon. I was scared that another relationship would end because of the physical distance. I was three hours away at college, and I wondered if our budding relationship would survive.

As my junior year of college started, I was scared and apprehensive. Kin and I had promised each other that we would find a way to make our relationship work even though we would be a three-hour drive away from each other. The first few weeks were busy. I was getting used to my class schedule and working part-time at a local daycare center in Sheboygan.

Kin and I saw each other once a month. I would usually drive home on Friday evenings after work and see Kin on Friday night and Saturday. It was very difficult for me to leave on Sunday afternoons, because I knew I wouldn't see Kin for another four weeks!

Throughout the winter months, Kin and I called each other at least twice a week. His voice on the other end of the line made me feel loved even though we were so far apart. As Christmas approached, I was excited and relieved that Kin and I would be sharing some quality time together.

The holidays were very busy that year. I spent Christmas Eve with my family and then dashed off so I could spend time with Kin and his family. It was nice to be with Kin again, and it was extremely hard for me to leave at the end of a relaxing evening.

As the school year progressed, Kin and I continued to see each other as much as my schedule would allow. I was taking fifteen credit hours, so I had plenty of schoolwork to keep me busy. I also worked part-time, so I had very little time to myself. However, our relationship seemed to grow stronger despite our distance from each other.

Finally, the academic year ended, and I was extremely happy to be heading back to my hometown. I could spend more time with Kin and get to know him better.

The first few weeks of summer were busy and I was happy. I was working at a daycare center about forty minutes from my parents' house. I was awake very early to work the 6:30 a.m. to 2:00 p.m. shift. I really enjoyed working with the children. Kin and I saw see each other in the evenings and spent as much time as we could together on the weekends.

Chapter 12

Summer Blues

S ometime toward the middle of June, my relationship with Kin changed. I felt being together for more than a year was terrific, but I wanted a long-term commitment. I was ready to get engaged. Kin, on the other hand, was very reluctant to ask me to marry him. He was content with our relationship as it was and didn't want to make any changes. We talked about the future and our dreams. He was also hesitant about having children, and I wanted to be a mother and wife someday soon.

After many hours of talking and some tears, Kin and I decided to go our separate ways.

The rest of the summer of 1999 was boring and lonely at best. I missed being with Kin and going out with him on weekends. This was the first time in eight years that I wasn't in a steady relationship. I hated being alone. I wanted to share the special moments in my life with someone.

Chapter 13

Blind Date

At the end of August, I was getting ready to return to college, and I remembered that my minister had asked if I would be willing to meet a nice guy from the congregation. When my minister had first approached me about dating this gentleman, I was dating Kin at the time, so I told her I was unavailable. Now I was single and wanted some companionship during my senior year at Lakeland College. So I gathered my courage and wrote a note to my minister and explained that I was interested in meeting the guy she had mentioned earlier.

The last few weeks of summer vacation went by quickly. One of my bosses at the daycare center set me up on a blind date with a guy she and her fiancé knew. I figured meeting the guy wouldn't hurt anything since I hadn't heard from my minister or the guy from Saron Church.

On a Thursday evening, I met Kurt. He was a nice guy and seemed interested in talking to me. After our first date, he asked for my phone number and I excitedly gave it to him without another thought.

As the last week of summer vacation approached, Kurt asked me out on a date. We went on a hike, which was fine, except I had not dressed for the occasion and was wearing some flimsy sandals that hurt my feet. I remember Kurt apologizing for not telling me in advance what we were doing. For me, I thought this was just typical guy stuff. In my experience, the guy almost never told me what or where we were going on a date.

During my separation and divorce, I had picked up the nasty habit of smoking. My previous boyfriends had also been smokers. However, Kurt wasn't a smoker and I didn't smoke around him for fear that he would call it quits with me right from the start. My intuition told me that not telling him I was a smoker was the wrong thing to do. I so wanted Kurt to like me that I thought this one little bad habit wouldn't matter that much.

The following weekend, I drove home for Labor Day. Kurt and I wanted to spend time together, and he still had no idea that I was a smoker. As we were talking on Sunday evening, I finally told Kurt that I smoked. I will never forget the look of disappointment and shock when I told him this. Kurt and I parted ways on Monday morning, and he had mentioned that he might come visit me at college on one of his bicycle trips in a few weeks.

Chapter 14

Conflict of Interest

Monday evening, as I was unpacking and relaxing, I got a call from David, the guy my pastor had mentioned. I was surprised and taken a little off guard, because I wasn't expecting David to call me. He sounded like a nice enough guy on the phone. In the back of my mind, I was thinking about Kurt and the weekend we had just spent together. *What was I supposed to do now?* Reluctantly, I told David that I was seeing someone else, and I didn't think going out with him was a good idea. David was very understanding, and I felt bad for him when we ended our first telephone conversation.

No sooner had I hung up with David than I received a phone call from Kurt. He said he didn't want to lead me on and we shouldn't see each other anymore. What the hell was this about? The guy had bought me flowers and spent the night with me, but I guess that meant more to me than it did to him. I hung up the phone and let out a deep sigh of disappointment and despair. *What was I supposed to do now?* I had just let David down, and I felt like a complete idiot for trusting Kurt enough to think that we could have a relationship.

I asked my roommate for advice, and she thought that I should call David back. But I didn't have his phone number. *Think, Kathy, think. How can you get David's number? Oh, of course, from the minister who had wanted to introduce us in the first place.* I sucked up every ounce of pride I had left and gave my minister a call.

She gave me David's number without questioning me, and then I quickly called David before I lost all my nerve. David answered the phone and appeared wary about my call. I explained that the other guy had broken up with me, and I would really like to go out with him. David asked me if I was sure about going out on a date, and I reassured him that I was willing to try a date. So we made plans to go out to dinner on Friday.

Chapter 15

First Date with David

As that Friday evening approached, I was nervous and excited. That afternoon I was anxious as I waited for the last of the parents to arrive and pick up their children from daycare. *Why did this parent always have to be late?* By the time I got back to my apartment, I found myself rushing around trying to get ready before David showed up for our date. Fortunately, my roommates were not home at the time so they weren't there to witness my nervous frenzy of activity.

After changing clothes several times, I finally decided on an outfit and finished getting ready. I heard the doorbell ring just as I put the final touches of my makeup on. I rushed to answer the door. Inside I felt like a nervous wreck, but on the outside, I was trying desperately to be calm, cool, and collected. David had a shy smile and looked genuinely happy to meet me.

I remember our first date so well. We went to a local restaurant for dinner. I don't remember eating the fish that I ordered, but I do remember telling David that I wasn't much of a meat eater. Then I realized I was telling a farmer that I disliked meat! Oh, how stupid could I get? But David was so great about my blunder. He said, "So I guess you are just gagging on that fish right now." I reassured him that I wasn't, and the conversation continued along very easily.

The drive back to my on-campus apartment was too short, at least for me. All the while David was driving, I kept thinking, *I don't want this date to end. How am I going to keep this date going?* So at the last minute, as David was parking the car in the school parking lot, I suggested that I give him a tour of the college campus. Now, what I was thinking I don't know. How much can you really see in the dark? I didn't care as long as I could prolong our date for a little bit longer.

David walked patiently beside me as I pointed out the buildings and scenery around the campus. I finished walking around the circle of the campus and couldn't think of any other way to extend our first date. Then David asked if he could walk me to my door. Seriously, I thought I was in heaven. Where had this guy been all my life? I unlocked the door to my apartment and stood waiting for my heart to stop pounding. David asked if he could call me again sometime and I said yes. The smiles that radiated from both of our faces probably could have lit up the entire apartment that night.

Chapter 16

A Budding Relationship

The next months went by in a flurry of activity. I was going to school full-time, working part-time, and starting a new relationship with someone very special. How did I manage it all? God only knows, but I managed. I longed for the weekends to last just a little longer so I could spend more time with David. Our relationship was blossoming into a friendship. David and I were both considerate of each other's feelings and the prior hurt we had endured from past relationships.

I don't remember the exact date, but I do remember that we were driving home from brunch after church one Sunday when suddenly David looks at me and says, "I think I'm falling in love with you. No, I *know* that I am falling in love with you."

My heart was singing and my mind was racing. I was having the same feelings, but David voiced them before I did! I also remember closing the door to my apartment that afternoon and feeling so loved and accepted for who I was and for who I was striving to be. I had never had this feeling before.

During my fall break from college, David asked if I would like to go look for appliances with him. I thought this was a strange request since I did not intend to tell him how to spend his money, especially on appliances. Earlier, David had told me that he would be moving into the house that his parents had rented for many years. He said this was the first time he felt like he needed a place of his own and a place he could share with me. Once again, I felt like the center of his universe, the most important thing in his life, and this awesome feeling truly made me grow to love David more.

Chapter 17

Falling in Love

The fall months scurried by, and I was quickly approaching the end of my first semester of my senior year. David and I had become a couple in every sense of the word. When I wasn't attending classes or working, I was spending time with him. This was difficult, because David was a farmer and I was a college student, but we managed. I was very unhappy when Christmas break rolled around, because we'd be apart for a while. David bought me a Harry Potter book and ruby earrings, which I never would have bought for myself. I don't even remember what I bought David that first Christmas. I'm guessing it was something inexpensive, as I was a poor college student!

I went home that Christmas wishing it were time to travel back to Sheboygan County so I could see David again. My parents had not yet met David, but I'm sure they were anxious to meet the guy who I couldn't stop talking about. Finally, my holiday break ended, and I traveled back to school anxious to see David again. I was scheduled to work part of my Christmas break, so I wouldn't be moping around the apartment when David and I weren't together.

I remember the first day or so of my winter break being extremely boring. The resort where I worked cut my hours, so I was barely working at all. What was I supposed to do with no money and a lot of time on my hands in the middle of winter? Watching television and listening to the radio got boring after the first few days. David came over almost every night, and I tried to get him to stay overnight, but morning comes very early for a farmer. Reluctantly, David would leave each evening to go home.

Chapter 18

New Year with New Love

I was excited about spending New Year's Eve with David. Neither of us wanted to go out and fight the party crowds, so I decided to make spaghetti and together we'd watch the ball drop in Times Square on television. Honestly, that doesn't sound overly romantic, but to me I couldn't think of any place I would rather be than at my on-campus apartment spending the evening with my boyfriend.

The new year brought even more work and responsibility for me. I began student teaching in January. I loved working with the first graders at the elementary school. My cooperating teacher was a terrific mentor, and I truly enjoyed going to my student teaching position each day. During this time, I was also taking a class at UW–Milwaukee.

Monday afternoons, after a full day of student teaching, I would travel to UW–Milwaukee for a document and design class. It wasn't what I had expected and certainly not the class I needed to replace the Advanced Composition class I was unable to take at Lakeland. Somehow, I managed to contribute enough to the class to pull off an A-minus.

Don't ask me how I did it, because I truthfully can't remember. All I know is that I don't want to be a publisher or an equivalent at any magazine or newspaper office.

The relationship that David and I had seemed to grow and blossom, unlike the cold winter weather that often hits Wisconsin. I enjoyed each weekend we spent together. There were a few times that I was disappointed because the winter weather made extra work for David on the farm.

I distinctly remember one Sunday morning when David called me an hour before church and said, "I don't think I'll be able to make it to church."

The alley scraper had broken down, and he didn't think he could get it fixed before church began. My disappointment must have come through quite clearly over the phone, because just as I was walking to the parking lot to dig my car out of the snow, David arrived looking a little disheveled, but he appeared just as happy to see me as I was to see him!

Chapter 19

More Responsibilities

In March, I started the second half of my student-teaching practicum. This time I was teaching middle school language arts. Unlike the first-grade students, I found I had to be a lot firmer in teaching and disciplining my middle school pupils. Once again, I was fortunate in that I had an excellent cooperating teacher who taught me how to deal with the challenges of teaching students in middle school. I was determined to make a good impression, and I arrived at school by 7:00 each morning.

As spring approached, I was anxious to leave the confines of college and begin a life with David. We had never really discussed moving in together or talked about what my plans would be once I graduated from college at the end of April. But the decision became very easy for me one night during my roommate's spring break. Because of my student-teaching schedule, I wasn't on spring break with the rest of the college students. Therefore, when my roommate came home at 9:00 p.m. one night and started being obnoxious and rowdy, I quickly packed a bag and took off for David's place.

I stormed into his house at a late hour and that surprised him. He looked at me and knew that I was extremely pissed off at something or someone. I told him I didn't want to talk about it. Slowly, I followed him upstairs and tried to relax enough to fall asleep. David didn't say much, but I finally confided in him that my roommate had been loud and irritating so I decided to stay the night with him. No discussion followed, but I do remember snuggling into David's arms and feeling the tension and anger slowly drain from my body. I think that was the most peaceful evening and good night's sleep I'd had in a long time!

The following week was my spring break. David and I discussed it, and we decided that I would stay with him at his house. It was almost as if we were married. I made supper every night, except on Mondays, because I still attended class at UW–Milwaukee. It felt so great to be spending extra time with David. By now, everyone considered us a couple. David and I were very comfortable with our relationship. We did everything together and it just felt right.

Chapter 20

Living Together

The last month of college before graduation went by quickly. David and I didn't really even discuss where I was going to live after I graduated. I remember gradually moving my clothes and personal belongings to his house. So by the time graduation rolled around, I had moved out of my on-campus apartment. We both felt this was the right decision.

When my parents and grandparents came for my graduation party, I announced that I was living with David. At this point, my parents didn't have much to say. I was thirty years old and had been supporting myself while finishing college. They weren't quick to offer advice this time around. I guess my parents figured out that their advice was only worth so much. However, my parents really liked David. They considered him a hardworking, honest guy. Somehow, they could tell that he would take care of me.

After graduation, I finished up with my student-teaching experience at the middle school. As June approached, I started looking for teaching jobs, and I filled out applications for every position that I could find. I felt discouraged, because most schools wanted someone with experience.

The summer of 2000, I took a job as a school-age teacher for KinderCare. They had a summer program, and I thought this would be good experience. The summer went by quickly. Part of my job was supervising the children when we went on field trips. That summer we went to the Milwaukee Zoo, Miller Park, and Chuck E. Cheese's. It was good experience, but I knew that this was not what I wanted to do the rest of my life.

The end of summer approached and I was discouraged because I hadn't heard from any of the school districts that had job offerings. I had one interview midsummer, but that didn't work out. At the end of August, I had an interview to teach at a private school in Fond du Lac. I enjoyed the interview very much and thought I had done really well. Finally, I received a phone call asking me if I wanted the position. Of course! Who was I to turn down my first full-time teaching position? I was hired as a fourth-grade teacher at a Catholic school. I was excited and nervous to start my new job right after Labor Day.

Chapter 21

First-Time Teacher

My first teaching position started out really well. I enjoyed the class of fourteen fourth graders, and I felt they were warming up to me as well. The first few weeks I was a strict disciplinarian. Each time one of the students misbehaved, they had to answer to me. But as the weeks continued, my classroom management style changed. I was frustrated having to reprimand the same students repeatedly for the same misbehaviors.

As Christmas approached, I felt like my teaching job was all about disciplining certain students in my class. I didn't feel like I was teaching them at all. The administrator of the consolidation of schools pulled me aside one day and told me that I needed to let one parent know each time her child misbehaved in class. I told the administrator that I would do this; however, in the back of my mind, I thought I would spend more time on the telephone with this student's mom than actually teaching.

Chapter 22

Making It Work

As Christmas approached, I longed to spend more time with David. We had been living together for eight months, and I already felt like we were a couple. One evening just after supper, I thought David was acting strange. He seemed nervous and preoccupied with something. As we were sitting on the couch during our quiet evening at home, he pulled a small box out from under the couch. He opened the box and said, "Kathy, do you think we can make it together?"

I was shocked and excited. The ring sparkled, and I wanted to see it on my finger, so I asked David to place it there. Then he asked, "Kathy, will you marry me?" I instantly said yes. I knew David was my soul mate, and I wanted to spend the rest of my life with him.

That evening we talked about the wedding, and we set the date for October 6, 2001. I had no idea how much planning and money went into a wedding celebration. I was on cloud nine and rode that cloud of excitement for the next several days.

As the new year approached, the student misbehaviors increased in the classroom. I felt I was not getting through to many of the students. Once again, the administrator took me aside and said that she had received complaints from several parents regarding my classroom management techniques. I was completely frustrated with the entire situation, and I anxiously awaited the end of the school year. When the administrator asked if I would renew my contract at the end of the school year, I told her I most likely would not.

Chapter 23

Leaving My Job

One late afternoon in February, the administrator came into my classroom. I was just finishing the school day. She told me this would be the hardest thing she had ever had to do. I looked at her and knew what was coming. I was asked to leave my teaching position immediately. I could send the administrator a letter of resignation, and she would accept it and put it in my file.

Looking back, I chalk this teaching position up to lack of experience. I have learned a lot since then. First, I have no desire to teach at a private school again. Second, I need to maintain a consistent and constant set of expectations and rules in my classroom. Third, I am perfectly happy substitute teaching at this time, so I can spend more time with my family.

David was so supportive when he heard the news. He said he didn't blame me for losing my teaching job. He just held my hand and told me he was sorry that I had lost my job. In bed that evening, I cried as David held me. He told me he didn't know what to say. All I really needed was his comforting arms, his reassurance, and his support.

The next few days I kept busy going to three of the area school districts. I filled out application forms so that I could substitute teach in each of the districts. I had never received my official teaching license so when it came to providing a copy of it to each district I was at a loss.

I called the Department of Public Instruction and inquired about my teaching license. The person on the other end of the phone told me it had never been printed or sent to me! I found this impossible to comprehend. How could a facility responsible for teaching licenses be so careless in handling such documents? My license finally arrived in the mail later that week, and I was relieved to have the certificate in my possession.

Chapter 24

Substitute Teaching

O nce my paperwork was in place at each of the school districts, I began to receive those early morning phone calls that many people despise. But I knew each call meant work, and I was determined to make the most of a crappy situation. So each day I would scramble out of bed and get ready to head to another sub job at one of the local schools.

That summer, I again took a job as a school-age teacher for KinderCare. I wanted to help make money so David and I could pay for our wedding, a beautiful wedding I had always dreamed of having. As the summer months passed, I went through all the preliminary wedding plans. I bought my dress, had it altered, and ordered the cake. We even went to marriage counseling sessions with our ministers.

As any bride and groom can tell you, preparations for a wedding seem endless, and David was terrific. He called to see if the church was available, made arrangements for the reception hall, and hired a disc jockey. I was excited and more than a little nervous when it came to planning such a big wedding.

The first time I got married, it was a very small affair. A Baptist minister I hardly knew performed the ceremony. Two of my ex-husband's close friends were our witnesses. It was a very simple, inexpensive ceremony, and not the wedding I had dreamed about having when I was a little girl.

Now we were planning a wedding with at least 150 guests. Most of my family was coming from out of town, and I was extremely excited to host relatives that I hadn't seen in quite some time.

Chapter 25

Our Wedding

The weather on our wedding day was gloomy and cold. The beautiful clear skies I had envisioned were nowhere to be found. As our friend Deb did my hair for the wedding, I prayed silently that the weather would improve. But as the morning wore on, the skies began to get darker and darker. So much for a sunny wedding day!

As I prepared for the ceremony, I thought back to the time David and I had spent together. This was it, the happiest day of my life. Yes, I had been married before, but it didn't feel anything like this. I couldn't wait to start the rest of my life with the man whom I loved and adored more than anything else in this world.

My brother started to sing the prelude just before the ceremony was about to start. As I stood waiting to walk down the aisle, a wave of nervousness hit me full tilt. I was shaking and my dad told me to calm down. I'm sure it was easy for him to say even though all eyes were on me. I don't enjoy being the center of attention, and my wedding day was no exception. However, once I reached the altar and looked into David's eyes, the nervous tension disappeared, and all I could think about was becoming Mrs. David Depping.

Pastor Jim gave a wonderful sermon about how it was the right time and the right place in our lives for us to be married. We had both been through some hard times, but we were ready to face the good and bad times together as husband and wife.

At our reception, I think I was glowing and feeling once again on cloud nine. I remember David saying, "You don't know what you've gotten yourself into." Truthfully, I had no idea what being a farmer's wife meant, but at that moment, I didn't care. I was happy, in love, and looking forward without any regrets.

Chapter 26

Trying to Start a Family

David and I settled into a comfortable routine. I was still subbing for three school districts and keeping very busy. There is always work to do on a farm, and the fall and winter months were no exception. David used the winter months to fix machinery inside the shed or catch up on other odd jobs around his parents' house or our own home.

Since we were a mature couple, we mutually decided that we would try to start a family right away. I went off birth control after we were married in October, but as the winter months went by, nothing happened. I became discouraged and frustrated. What could I be doing wrong? Why wasn't I getting pregnant? I tried to console myself and kept hoping that it would happen.

It was difficult to see other people who I was close to getting pregnant and having children. I tried very hard to be happy for them, but deep down I envied them and wanted desperately to have a child of my own.

David and I kept trying to get pregnant but were unsuccessful. Fertility becomes a big issue when you are unable to conceive naturally. However, David was very supportive and wanted to make me happy no matter the cost. David would sacrifice his own health and well-being to make everyone else around him happy and content.

As the months continued to drift by with no luck, I thought about checking into a fertility specialist. David wasn't ready for that yet, and I truthfully thought we could try to conceive a child naturally for just a little longer. But before we knew it, two years had gone by and we still weren't pregnant.

Chapter 27

Fertility Treatments

I talked to my gynecologist about trying alternative ways to get pregnant. He mentioned first having David's sperm count evaluated. Well, let me tell you, I had no idea what that entailed. After the tests were done, my doctor mentioned trying a procedure called IUI—intrauterine insemination. Not to oversimplify the procedure, but what happens is a sperm sample is taken and put through a cleaning process. Then the cleaned sperm is injected into the female during ovulation, which is a very short time frame during a woman's monthly cycle. Then for at least half an hour, you lay on an exam table while you wait for the sperm to do its job—fertilize the egg!

Sounds simple, right? Well, not exactly. First, I had to determine when I was ovulating. I have never been that in-tune with my body before, so this was difficult for me. Once I determined when I was ovulating, David would have to get a sperm sample to the clinic at least thirty minutes before I was scheduled to be there for the IUI.

Scheduling these types of procedures was time consuming and not the romantic, intimate way of conceiving a child, but David and I were determined to have a child of our own.

After four failed attempts with the IUI, my gynecologist told me there was nothing else he could do for me, but he did offer us hope. There was a fertility specialist in Green Bay that had an excellent success rate with IVF—in vitro fertilization.

Chapter 28

The IVF Journey

David and I discussed in vitro fertilization at great length. After some tears and many long nights of praying, we decided to go ahead and see what this process entailed. The well-respected specialist we were going to see was in demand, so it took almost a month before we could get a consultation. The day we met the doctor, I knew everything would be fine.

Not only did this doctor offer hope to someone who thought she would never have a child, but also he was also willing to get to know me as a person, as a woman who longed to have a child. From the moment I walked out of that first meeting with Dr. X, I knew that whatever challenges David and I faced, we would make it through them together.

The first step of the IVF process was extensive physical workups done on both of us. I hated having another pap exam and more blood drawn, but I knew it would be worth it if we were able to have a baby. David also went through a battery of tests. We anxiously awaited the results of the tests and wondered what the next step would be in the process.

At our next visit with Dr. X, we discussed the results of the test. David's sperm count was extremely low, and he would most likely not impregnate me in a natural way. However, there is a procedure called ICSI—intracytoplasmic sperm injection. This procedure involves injecting a single sperm directly into a mature egg to achieve fertilization. The fertilized egg is then kept in a laboratory for three days until it has grown to eight blastomeres. The cells are then implanted back into the woman's womb in hopes they will attach to the uterus and the woman becomes pregnant.

This sounded great! Sign us up! When do we begin? Questions ran through our minds as we patiently listened to the doctor. We had no idea what we were getting into even though the doctor specifically told us there was a chance that the procedure wouldn't work. He said we would either start back at the beginning or give up on the idea of getting pregnant altogether. But from our first meeting, I knew Dr. X was determined to give it his best to help us fulfill our dream of becoming parents.

The IVF process is complicated and hard to explain, but from my point of view, the procedure was well worth the risk and expense. The first thing the doctor does is take complete control of your menstrual cycle. You are given hormones that are supposed to increase the number of eggs that you produce during your cycle. Then you are given progesterone and estrogen to help your body get ready for pregnancy. I'm sure I am oversimplifying a highly scientific process.

I remember going in several times each week and having blood drawn. This was to determine how much of a hormone injection I would receive on any given day. It became very time consuming and my arms were bruised from the many needle pokes.

Finally, Dr. X said that my hormone levels were good and that I had four or five good eggs that they would retrieve for the ICSI procedure. The doctor told us that ICSI was a good option since David's sperm count was so low. I was nervous and scared. What would the retrieval feel like? The egg retrieval was scheduled for 8:00 a.m., which meant David had to get up very early to do the milking and the chores before we headed to Green Bay for the procedure.

Chapter 29

The Retrieval and Implantation

Most mornings, David was usually awake and out of the house early to do chores. But the morning of the retrieval, I was also awake. Even though I knew it was super early, I just couldn't seem to fall back asleep. My mind was working overtime trying to imagine how the procedure would feel.

When we arrived at the fertility clinic, I was apprehensive and nervous. I knew the doctor would put me under anesthesia for the procedure, but I still didn't know quite what to expect. As I was given the sedative, David sat patiently by my side and tried to reassure me that everything would be fine. Despite his best efforts, I was still nervous and scared. I guess this is to be expected when you undergo any type of procedure, even if it is very unlikely something bad will happen.

I don't remember anything that went on in the operating room. The first thing I asked when I came out of the anesthesia was, "How many eggs did they retrieve?" David told me at least three times that they had retrieved four eggs, but I guess I was too groggy to comprehend what he said the first time.

David sat quietly by my bedside while we waited for the effects of the anesthesia to wear off. The doctor came and checked on me several times and told us that he had retrieved four eggs. I felt excited and a little doubtful. Would this be a significant number of eggs to fertilize and give us one or two healthy embryos? David was so gentle and patient as we sat and waited to be released so we could drive home.

Just before we were ready to leave, the doctor came and explained that for the next three days the embryology specialist would watch the cells and see which ones would be viable to implant back into my uterus. This still sounded foreign and unbelievable to me. Whatever happened to the old-fashioned way of getting pregnant? I still couldn't believe that this was a conceivable way of getting pregnant. We left the clinic feeling hopeful and exhausted.

The next day, Dr. X called and told me that four embryos had fertilized! I was so happy but also still scared about the process of getting pregnant this way. In another two days, we would be back at the clinic for embryo implantation. Implantation occurs when the embryos are put back into the uterus by another surgical procedure.

As the day of implantation arrived, I was again too excited to sleep. I had so many things running through my head that I felt like I could burst! Would the procedure hurt? Would I be able to handle three days of bed rest in order to ensure that the implantation had a chance to work? So many mixed emotions—excitement, apprehension, and a little disbelief—still wandered into my thoughts.

I remember arriving at the clinic and the staff being supersensitive to our needs. Dr. X told us he would implant three embryos into my uterus. The fourth embryo had fragmented, and the chance of it being a normal embryo was unlikely. A shot of Demerol relaxed me, but I would be awake during the implantation procedure. Finally, I was wheeled into the examination room and the process began. Dr. X talked to me the entire time. He told me what he was doing as he went along. Then I felt the most incredible cramping pain ever! I'm not sure what it was, but I was willing to endure just about anything to become pregnant.

After the embryos were implanted into my uterus, we had to wait an hour just to make sure that things were looking okay. I wasn't looking forward to spending three days on bed rest; I need to be doing something all the time. I'm constantly in motion, and I knew bed rest would be a very tough thing for me to do. Again, I knew that this was all to help ensure that I became pregnant.

Finally, we were allowed to leave the clinic. The ride home was a bit uncomfortable, as I had to lie in the backseat of the Buick. Once we got home, David settled me into a recliner, which would be my throne for the next three days. I was so tired from the procedure and from waking up early that morning that I slept the rest of the afternoon.

Chapter 30

Bed Rest and Restlessness

The next three days were the longest three days of my life! I am the type of person who always needs to be doing something, so being confined to a chair was very difficult. I thought about my dream of becoming a mother and having an infant, so that kept me going throughout the three days of required bed rest.

The first day I watched movies and visited with my friend Sandy. The time passed by quickly with her company, and I was happy to talk with her. David spent some time with me, but he also had a farm to run and chores to do. He would come home for lunch and check on me, and then he would come home again after he finished the evening chores. The second day was a little tough to handle.

It was a rainy Memorial Day weekend, and I was bored out of my mind. I read, watched television, and napped, but the time seemed to crawl by. David was such a good sport about the whole thing and tried hard to keep me entertained when he was home. By the end of the third day, I was going stir-crazy. I couldn't wait to get up and move around. The thought of even going for a short walk outdoors sounded like a little piece of heaven on earth.

Tuesday I was finally able to move around again. I felt a little weak and sore, but I was extremely glad to get up and out of the house. We would have to wait until the first week of June to see if I was pregnant. The waiting game was the hardest thing to take. Each day I prayed that God would be kind and allow David and me to have a child. My faith and a strong desire to be a mother kept me going as we waited for the day when I would have a pregnancy test.

Those of you who have never had to go through fertility treatments are extremely lucky. In order for an IVF cycle to be successful, a woman is given hormone shots to increase the number of eggs that she produces each month. Let me tell you, the shots given twice daily are no picnic. Your butt and thighs are so bruised that they ache miserably. But with each shot I got, I kept telling myself that this would be worth it when and if I got pregnant.

Chapter 31

The Pregnancy Test

On June 9, 2004, I woke up early. I was excited and nervous to find out the results of the pregnancy test. A simple blood test can determine if you are pregnant or not. The drive to Aurora BayCare seemed to go by quickly. Maybe because this was the day we would find out if the IVF procedure had worked. I was in and out of the clinic in less than thirty minutes, because drawing blood takes almost no time at all.

The drive home was filled with eagerness and worry. What would the test reveal? Would I be pregnant or would we have to consider giving up our dream of becoming parents? I arrived home and David was waiting for me.

David and I ate lunch in nervous anticipation. I kept looking at the clock and wishing someone would call with my blood test results. Finally, at 1:15 p.m. a nurse called. I was pregnant!

She instructed me to return to the fertility clinic in two days for more blood work.

Tears of joy rolled down my cheeks when I told David. God had answered our prayers. We both knew that this was the first step in my pregnancy, and I was determined to stay fit and deliver a healthy baby.

David and I decided to keep my pregnancy a secret until the end of my first trimester. We didn't want to have to explain anything if I happened to miscarry early on during the pregnancy. It was hard to keep such terrific news secret, especially from my parents and close friends.

The summer began rainy and wet. David was stressed because things weren't going well on the farm. One of the cows died after suffering a twisted uterus and losing her calf. Then another cow died. These things sometimes happen, but it is a financial loss when you lose a few cows in a small herd. Because of the wet weather, the milking cows had not been out to pasture and it was already June 25!

I felt like I should be doing something to help David, but I also knew that he didn't want me to get too close to the cows in case one of them would happen to kick me. We had been through so much for me to get pregnant that we didn't want any little mishap to jeopardize my pregnancy.

David was sensitive to my needs and kept reminding me that I should take it easy and try not to do too much. Since I can't sit still for too long, his advice was extremely hard to follow. I knew all he wanted was for me to stay well and for us to have a healthy baby in February.

Chapter 32

My Pregnancy Experiences

On June 28, 2004, David and I traveled to the fertility clinic for my ultrasound. On the drive, I began to feel nauseated and sick. This feeling hadn't happened yet, and it was a new symptom of pregnancy for me. When the doctor placed the ultrasound probe on my flat belly and began to move it around, I became even more excited. A tiny flicker of a heartbeat indicated there was one baby. It was truly reassuring to see the heartbeat on the monitor.

I became a very happy, yet sick, pregnant woman. Why physicians and others call it morning sickness is beyond me. I felt sick all day! I tried to eat saltines, and I followed other remedies, but most of them didn't work. There were some days when I just laid on the couch and slept or tried to wish the nausea away. I never threw up; it was more dry heaves, and my dislike of saltines has carried over since then.

Going through IVF made me appreciate how precious being pregnant can be. In order to sustain the pregnancy, I continued with progesterone shots until July 30. I was so excited to be free of the daily injections that I'd been taking for months. I also loved getting the ultrasound pictures of the baby every other week. It was amazing to hear the heartbeat and see the tiny feet and umbilical cord.

My scheduled visits to Dr. X's office continued until the beginning of August. After the first trimester, the specialist sends you back to your regular gynecologist. I was a little sad to leave the friendly staff I had grown accustomed to seeing during the past several months. But I was also looking forward to being cared for by my regular doctor who I knew would take very good care of me.

Chapter 33

Health Issues for David

As I began my second trimester, I began to feel more energetic and less nauseated. I made a conscious effort to eat small snacks and healthy foods.

During the first part of September, David started to feel ill. On occasion, his colitis would flare up, and he would feel nauseated and have terrible stomach pains. I did not think too much about the flare-ups, because David occasionally had them; they would go away, and he'd feel better.

However, this time he seemed more tired and more uncomfortable. He was never the kind of person to complain about aches and pains, so when he went to see a doctor, I knew he wasn't feeling well.

David saw one of the family practice doctors for a check-up, and she suggested that he make an appointment with his gastrointestinal specialist. However, when David called in September to set up an appointment, he was told the doctor was on vacation for several weeks.

So David grinned and bore the discomfort. We celebrated our third wedding anniversary by going out for a pizza. Nothing too extravagant, but it was a quiet and romantic dinner for the both of us.

Chapter 34

My Brother's Wedding

The weekend of October 9, we traveled to Merrill for my brother's wedding. I sensed David wasn't feeling well. He was very quiet, and he rested at my parents' house while I took care of some last-minute details before the rehearsal dinner.

The weekend weather was beautiful for October. I recall it was seventy degrees and sunny and made for gorgeous wedding pictures. I specifically asked the photographer to take a picture of David and me, as we didn't have a recent photo of us together.

David and I left the wedding reception about 11:00 p.m. We were both tired and wanted to get some rest before we traveled back to Plymouth on Sunday. Sunday morning we stayed at my parents' for a little while. David held Brandon, our nephew, who was a cute, healthy five-month-old boy. I enjoyed watching David interact with Brandon and thought about what it would be like for him to interact with our own child in four more months.

Chapter 35

Unexpected ER Visit

After our weekend in Merrill, David still wasn't feeling well. He had been to see a family practice doctor who put him on antibiotics for thrush that made David's mouth extremely sore. I took him to the ER, because he was having such bad pains in his abdomen. Each time we saw a doctor, we would mention that David had colitis, and this was most likely a flare-up of some kind. The doctors would draw some blood and do a few tests, but found nothing abnormal. It was extremely frustrating. David still felt tired and weak and no one had answers for us.

David woke me up around 3:00 a.m. on Sunday, October 17, 2004. He said he was in a lot of pain and very uncomfortable. Since David isn't one to complain, I knew he didn't feel well. As I quickly dressed, David said that maybe we should wait, because the pain wasn't too awful. I told him that if it was bad enough to wake me up, we were going to the emergency room.

As I drove to the ER, I could tell David was in a lot of pain. His face was pale, and he cringed every time I went over a bump. I was extremely concerned at what was making him so uncomfortable and causing him so much pain. When we arrived at the ER, I helped David into the entrance and went to park the car.

David's pain seemed to increase as we sat waiting for the ER doctor. Again, we mentioned that David had colitis, but this time he was in a tremendous amount of agony. The doctor ordered a shot of morphine to help ease the pain. As the minutes passed into an hour, I could tell the medicine was doing nothing to alleviate David's awful ache. I asked the nurse on duty if David could have more medicine, but I felt like she was blowing me off. She said more pain medicine could cause breathing problems. The doctor evaluated David's symptoms and decided to perform a CAT scan of his abdomen. The test results were unclear, and the doctor claimed he couldn't find the cause of David's unbearable pain.

I was anxious and mad by this time. We had arrived at the ER about 3:30 a.m. and now it was around 5:00 or 6:00 a.m., and we still had no answers. In fact, with each hour that passed, his symptoms worsened. At one point, David asked to be knocked out, because he just couldn't stand the pain anymore! I sat by his side feeling helpless and furious. The doctor didn't offer comfort or seem to understand how bad David was suffering from the intensifying pain!

Chapter 36

Emergency Surgery

Around 6:30 a.m., the ER doctor decided it was time to admit David to the hospital. We had arrived almost four hours ago, and we still had absolutely no idea why David felt so ill. I remember a gurney being wheeled up to the second floor of the hospital. As the nurse took David's vitals and inquired about his symptoms, she also asked the name of his physician. I told her it was Dr. Z. The nurse then told me the doctor didn't accept calls on the weekend and couldn't be called to the hospital. I was livid! How could a doctor not be available for his patients? What were we supposed to do now?

At around 7:30 or 8:00 a.m., the on-call doctor came into David's room. Immediately, she could tell that David was in tremendous pain and ordered more morphine. She told us that she was going to order another scan of David's abdomen and GI tract to determine what was going on. I sat impatiently waiting for the results while David moaned in pain.

After about thirty minutes, the on-call doctor came in and said the scan showed a tear in David's colon and large intestine! She was going to call in a surgeon immediately and consult with him about how to proceed with David's treatment.

After about an hour, the surgeon and the on-call doctor came in the room, both looking extremely concerned. The surgeon confirmed that David had a tear in his large intestine. He also explained that from the scan, it appeared as if David's entire large intestine was damaged, and depending on what he found during surgery, the large intestine may have to be removed. The surgeon went on to explain that David would wear a colostomy bag, which would empty the waste from his body. The bag would take the place of the job once done by his large intestine.

David looked to me for answers. What should we do? As far as I was concerned, surgery seemed the only option to keep my husband alive and from enduring extreme pain. So the staff prepped David for surgery. I gave him a kiss and prayed he would make it through surgery. We hoped we would get some answers soon.

Waiting for someone to have a surgical procedure is agonizing! I remember sitting in David's hospital room for a while, and then I went outside and called my parents to let them know what had happened. My parents were extremely concerned and said they would travel to Plymouth to help on the farm for a few days. I also called David's mom and told her what was going on. She sounded very worried for her son and told me to let her know how things progressed.

Minutes seemed to tick by so slowly. I waited anxiously from 1 p.m. until 3:55 p.m. for someone to tell me how the operation went. Finally, the surgeon came into David's room and told me that he had removed David's entire colon and large intestine. The diseased colon had spewed pus into David's body, which took more work to clean out.

For another hour, I waited while David remained in the recovery room. David's aunt Vernita came to sit with me for a while. She sat quietly and kept me company. Finally, David was wheeled into the hospital room. He was still very groggy from the anesthesia. The details are foggy, but I remember David talking a little bit to my brothers, Mark and Erik, when they arrived around 6:00 p.m. My parents arrived shortly after and tried to comfort David as well.

By seven o'clock that evening, I was physically and emotionally exhausted! It had been an extremely long day for David and me. I kissed David and told him I would return in the morning to see how he was doing. I spent most of the next day in the hospital with David. My parents decided to stay that week and help on the farm as much as they could.

Chapter 37

The Diagnosis

During this time, I was trying to complete my master's degree through UW–Oshkosh. I had two classes to complete before receiving my degree, and I was hoping to finish them before the baby was born. One of the classes involved research for my educational proposal on teacher mentoring programs. The other class was an online classroom management course, so I spent a lot of time on the computer.

Early Tuesday morning on October 19, I went to Manitowoc to interview two teachers before I went to visit David at the hospital. When I arrived at the hospital, I could sense that David was preoccupied. He told me he was glad that my mom was with me. David took a deep breath, and then told me that Dr. X had received the pathology reports from his surgery. The reports showed that David had cancer in his colon and that it had spread to the lymph nodes! The doctor wasn't sure if they had gotten all the cancer during surgery, but wanted to wait until David was stronger before starting any form of treatment.

I sat there facing the worst possible news ever! How had this happened? How does a fairly healthy man go from being a little sick to having colon cancer? What were we faced with now? The uncertainty and shock settled in, and my emotions took over and I cried, but I also believed in my heart that we could get through this together. God had given us a challenge, and it was something that would test our faith and love for each other. I had faith that David would beat this terrible disease and live to witness the birth of his daughter.

Chapter 38

Recuperating and Moving On

David had always been a go-getter, always on the move, and doing more work than the average guy probably should. So when he came home from the hospital on October 24, he felt he needed to be out in the barn, even if it was only to supervise. I knew better than to fight with him about this, because it was one battle I wouldn't win. He felt useful supervising and giving advice to my dad and the person we had milking the cows; this was preferable to feeling useless sitting around the house.

Our baby continued to grow and stay healthy despite the turmoil that David and I experienced each day. David was learning to adjust to wearing a colostomy bag and having to empty and change it every few days. The site of his incision drained a lot and kept us visiting the emergency room just to be certain he wasn't fighting an infection.

We made several trips to the doctor's office for David, one to have the staples removed from the incision area, and another that involved blood work to rule out postoperative infection or other complications.

One of our clinic visits was to get an ultrasound of the baby. This was one of the exciting and happy times in the midst of uncertainty and endless tests for David. As we sat together watching the technician roll the probe around my expanding belly, we marveled at the tiny hands, feet, and heartbeat! When the technician told us the baby was most likely a girl, we were both elated. We looked forward to the day when we would bring our little girl home and enjoy being parents.

Chapter 39

More Bad News

David was readmitted to the hospital after a CAT scan on November 5. The scan revealed some spots on David's liver, but the doctor didn't think they were cancerous. The next step was to treat the cysts on David's liver with IV antibiotics.

The previous week had been hectic. David's incision had drained constantly due to a pus pocket. The doctor opened the incision so it could drain and heal better. David commented that the incision had bled a lot the previous night, and the nurses' had to apply an uncomfortable pressure pack directly on the incision to get the bleeding to stop. I was grateful David had been in the hospital when this happened. He was well taken care of and could be monitored.

David had a PICC (peripherally inserted central catheter) line put in his arm on November 8. This allowed him to receive IV antibiotics at home for the next three weeks. During this time, the doctor could monitor him and see how the cysts on his liver responded to the antibiotics. I also learned how to flush his PICC line after each dose of antibiotics. I started feeling like a nurse, mainly because I was David's primary caregiver. However, I was willing and up for the challenge of being a caregiver, especially if it meant that David could be at home. We could spend time together as a family.

My pregnancy progressed. We experienced a whirlwind of doctor appointments; however, most of them were for David. I had an ultrasound done on November 17, and the technician told us we were having a girl. I think David was just as excited as I was. I also had an appointment with my OB doctor and I mentioned to him what was happening with David.

My doctor was very reassuring and told me that he knew of many people who had survived colon cancer.

Leading up to the Thanksgiving holiday, David started feeling ill again. The visiting nurse looked at David's incision site and thought it didn't look right. So on November 22, we went back to the hospital where David had yet another CAT scan.

The following day, David had an appointment with the surgeon to discuss the results of the scan. They were not promising. David's liver wasn't responding to the antibiotics that he had been taking for the past several weeks. So the surgeon suggested admitting David into the hospital so they could do a liver biopsy.

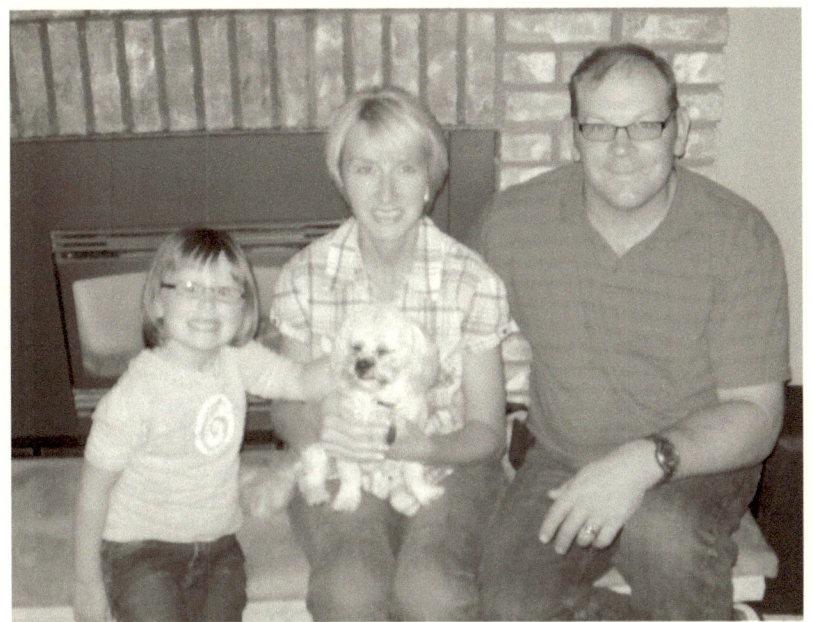

Anna, Kathy, Brandi (our dog), Ryan

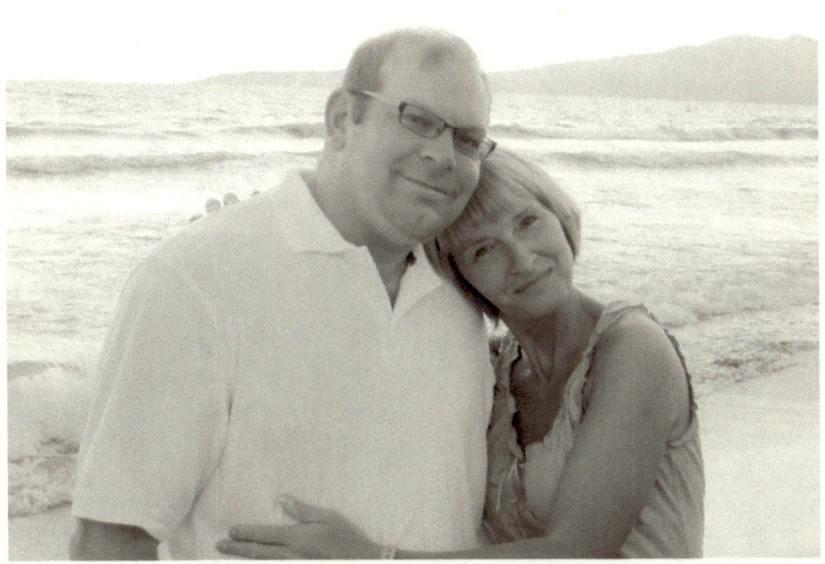

Ryan and Kathy (Mexico 2011)

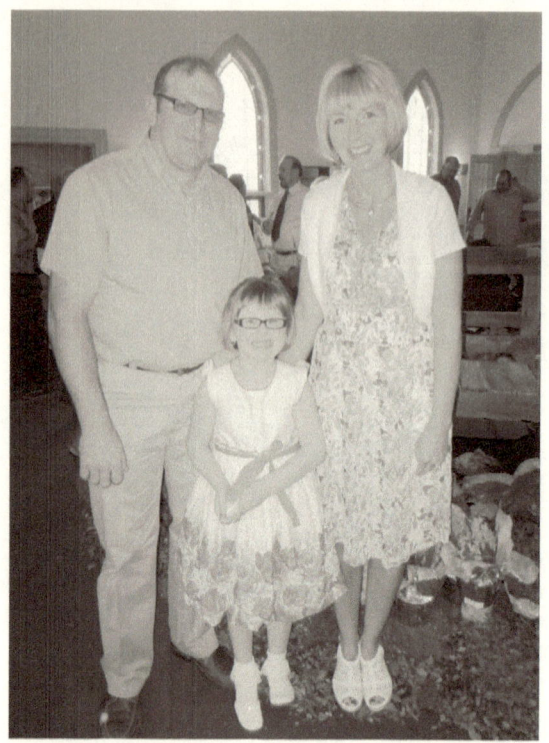

Ryan, Anna, Kathy (Easter 2011)

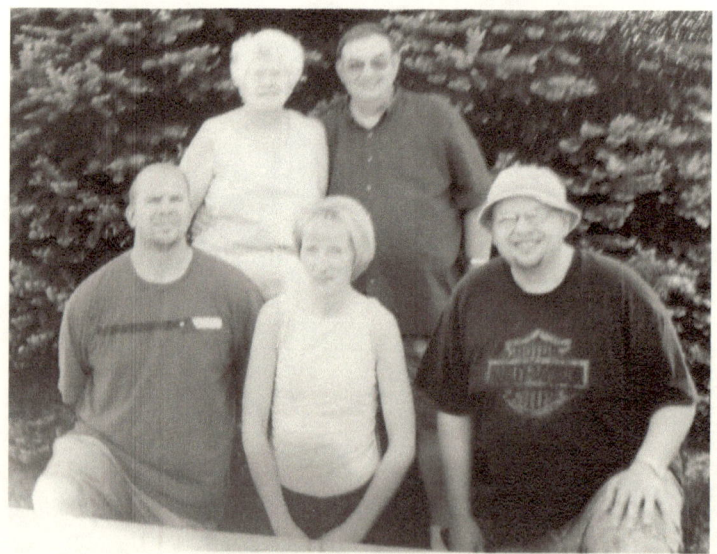

Front row: Erik, Kathy, Mark
Back row: Sonya, John

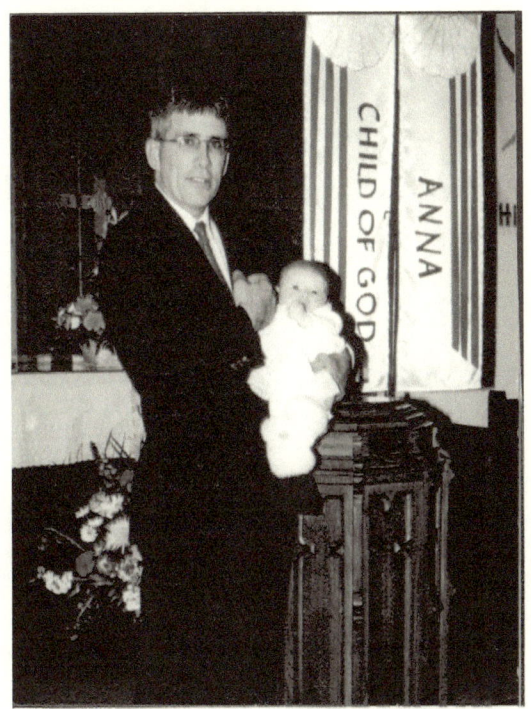

Brian and Anna (at Anna's baptism)

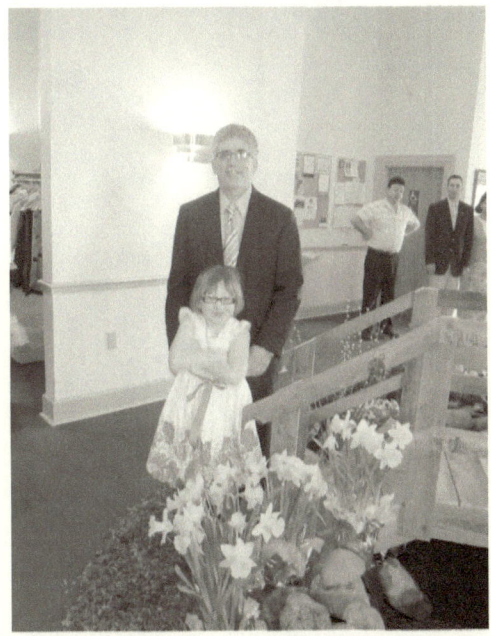

Brian and Anna (Easter 2011)

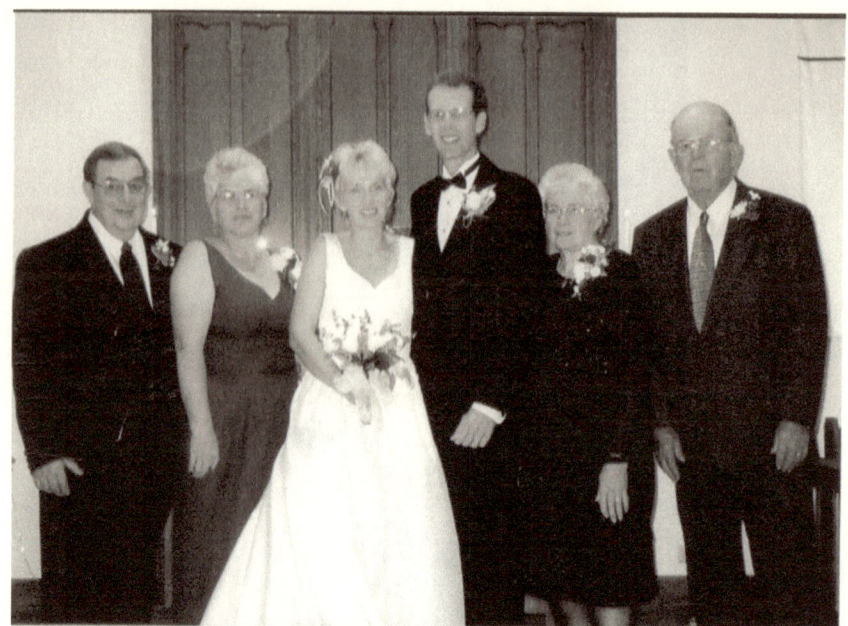

Left to right: John, Sonya, Kathy, David, Evelyn, Harold (at our wedding, October 2001)

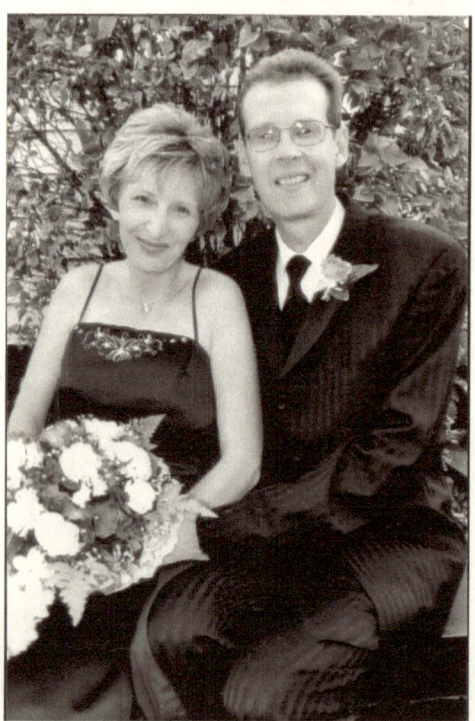

Kathy and David (at my brother's wedding, October 2004)

Chapter 40

Biopsy Complications

David's blood levels were so high on Tuesday that the doctor refused to do the biopsy. He feared David might bleed internally. Instead, David was given eight units of plasma to get his blood levels up. Now, I have no medical training, but in my gut, I knew something was terribly wrong. I kept thinking to myself that the cancer had spread to his liver. However, this was something I never spoke aloud about for fear my instincts might actually be true.

When I arrived at the hospital on Wednesday morning, the nurse was giving David his last unit of plasma. David's blood levels were checked again, and the doctor determined his blood levels were safe enough to proceed with the liver biopsy.

David was apprehensive about the biopsy and asked if it would be painful. The nurse assured him that he would be given a local anesthesia to lessen any pain. I waited anxiously as my husband was taken to radiology for the biopsy.

When David returned to his room, I could sense he was in a tremendous amount of pain. The nurse gave him a shot of morphine to comfort him. I stayed with David until about four that afternoon watching and hoping that he would be able to rest after the ordeal of his liver biopsy.

At around 7:30 that evening, I received a telephone call at home from one of the nurses taking care of David. She told me he was in terrible pain and going in for another CAT scan. I sensed a certain edge to her voice, one filled with concern and fear. She suggested I come to the hospital as soon as possible. I quickly got in my car and sped off not knowing what condition I would find my husband in this time.

When I arrived at the hospital, I rapidly made my way to the second floor. I found David struggling to get air and being wheeled to radiology for yet another CAT scan. David looked deathly pale and so uncomfortable. I felt helpless and sick to my stomach as I again waited for more results. David was taken immediately from radiology to the intensive care unit where he was monitored for his irregular breathing.

The surgeon on call that evening explained that David was bleeding into his lung. This caused a buildup of fluid and made it extremely difficult for him to breathe. They inserted a chest tube to drain the blood from David's chest cavity.

This occurred the evening before Thanksgiving 2004, and I was once again spending time in the hospital. David was in stable condition, but I wasn't about to leave the hospital for fear he might take another turn for the worse and die alone! This may sound horrific and pessimistic, but I was determined to be with him no matter what happened.

Chapter 41

A Bleak Prognosis

On Thanksgiving Day 2004, David remained in a stable but weak condition. The liver biopsy and subsequent bleeding in his chest cavity had left him extremely frail. I was grateful he was moved to ICU where he would receive one-on-one care. I kept thinking God had a purpose for us, but I just wasn't sure what it was and how it would be revealed. I tried to remain optimistic and hoped David's condition would improve so we could both enjoy the birth of our daughter in just two and a half months.

I grew accustomed to eating meals in the cafeteria. The Thanksgiving meal was very good considering it was hospital food. I was grateful to have somewhere to go that was away from the sterile, depressing hospital room that had become David's permanent place of residence during the past several weeks. The cafeteria was where I would let out a big sigh and try to relax even if for just half an hour.

Though David was extremely ill, he constantly worried about the baby and me. We never really discussed the possibility that he would die, because he didn't want to stress me out anymore than I already was. I think this was his way of protecting me from knowing just how serious his illness was. I found some comfort in believing that his condition would improve, and he would be well enough for the birth of his daughter in February.

Friday, November 26, will be one of those days I will remember for the rest of my life. It started out pretty normal. I arrived at the hospital around 9:00 a.m. and made my way to the ICU unit where David's room was. When I got there, I knew something was terribly wrong, because both of our ministers were there. David had a look of utter despair and disappointment. The first thing that entered my mind was, *Now what has gone wrong? What has happened?*

I searched David's eyes for an explanation. I sat in intense anguish listening while he began another cautious but sad story about his condition. The surgeon had received the pathology report from the liver biopsy. The report showed the cancer had spread to David's liver, and it was a very aggressive type of cancer. The prognosis was bleak, and the surgeon was certain David had no chance of survival. There was very little anyone could do for him at this time.

As tears streamed down my cheeks and sobs wracked my body, I tried to take in what David had just said. He had colon cancer, which had now spread to his liver. The liver cancer was very aggressive, and he didn't have a chance of survival.

Although the prognosis was bleak, I couldn't accept it without more answers. There had to be something that could be done for my husband, the most important person in my life! I was unwilling to accept the prognosis and admit defeat. Neither David nor myself considered ourselves quitters, and if he wasn't strong enough to fight this battle alone, then I sure as hell was going to do anything I could to help him put up the best fight possible. Sure, he may not survive this, but maybe there was some small chance that he would improve and be able to see his daughter being born. In my heart, I believe that is what we both hoped for and wanted.

My mind raced into overdrive. I asked someone to contact the head oncology nurse. I needed to speak to her right away. I needed answers that I felt were long overdue.

The oncology nurse walked into David's room looking concerned and appeared out of the loop. The oncology department hadn't been involved in David's treatment up until this point. The surgeon felt that David needed to recover from the initial surgery done on his colon before we could consider treatment for colon cancer.

The oncology nurse looked at David and then at me and said someone had better tell her what was going on. David couldn't articulate what was happening to him one more time, so I began the story about his condition. The oncology nurse listened with the patience and concern that I believe is required of nurses and doctors in the oncology field.

Then she told us she would call Dr. K and have him look at David's charts and X-rays. She said that as soon as Dr. K had a chance to review everything, he would come in and talk to us about the next step. As Stephanie, the oncology nurse, left the room, I was relieved yet worried that we would now find out the seriousness of David's condition. Would he live another week, another month? Realistically, I don't think anyone had that answer, but I needed to know for my own peace of mind, and I think David really wanted to know too.

Chapter 42

Oncologist on Board

After going through David's charts and X-rays, Dr. K came in and spoke with us for about an hour. From our initial meeting, I could tell Dr. K was hopeful, and he offered compassion and sympathy when many of the other medical professionals up until this point had not. Dr. K explained that David's cancer had indeed spread to his liver and that this type of cancer does spread at a rapid rate. Therefore, Dr. K wanted to try two chemotherapy drugs on David as soon as possible.

Dr. K was also very honest and told us there were no guarantees with the treatment, but that it might stop the cancer from progressing. The goal that we all hoped to achieve was for David to live long enough to see his daughter being born.

David's condition seemed like a roller coaster in motion. One day he was feeling a little better, and the next day he would take a turn for the worse. On November 28, I rushed to the hospital once again, because David's heartbeat was extremely fast. The doctor on call tried three times to shock David's heart back into a normal rhythm. After these failed attempts, they gave him medicine to help slow his heart rate. Thankfully, during the night David's heart rate decreased, and he was once again in stable condition.

Chapter 43

Cancer Treatments and Challenges

On Monday, David started his first round of chemotherapy drugs. First, he was given premeds to fight off nausea. All the chemo medicines had to be double-checked to assure that David was getting the proper treatment. I tried to remain optimistic and stay focused on being calm. My pregnancy meant the world to us and at that point, I didn't want to jeopardize going into preterm labor.

Each day David faced new challenges with his condition. He didn't have a will made up, and it bothered him that he might die without having his wishes met. So one morning we worked with the hospital social worker and filled out the power of attorney for health care papers. David felt better after completing the paperwork, because he knew his wishes would be in order, should he take a turn for the worse and die.

On December 2, David moved out of ICU and back to a room on the cancer unit of 2K. I helped him clean up, which was a major undertaking since he hadn't been out of bed for a week. I could tell the sponge bath, shaving, and brushing of his teeth wore David out, but he told me he felt a little better because he was clean.

Dr. X ordered an ultrasound of David's legs to see if there were any blood clots. David had swelling in his lower arms and legs, and the doctor was hoping to find out what was causing the swelling.

On December 7, one of the oncologists started David on pain patches. David was very uncomfortable, because it takes at least twelve hours for the full dose of pain meds to disperse through the patch. The occupational therapists and physical therapists arrived and had David sit at the edge of his bed. He was still swelling in his legs, arms, and abdomen area.

December 9 was a rainy, dreary day. One of David's friends was a nurse and spent extra time getting him cleaned up and bathed that day. His legs, arms, and private area were still swollen. I wish I could have made the pain and extra "stuff" just disappear, but realistically, I knew I couldn't. David was so frustrated, because he couldn't walk around and do things for himself. I knew he was doing the best he could to get stronger, because he wanted to see his daughter being born.

Chapter 44

Arrangements to Sell Our Farm

During this time, David realized his illness was terminal. After considerable discussion and worry, he decided it was time to sell the cattle. David was very concerned because other people were now running the farm, and he didn't want this to continue. This was a very difficult decision on his part, as the farm had been in his family for more than a hundred years. But after talking it over with his father, Harold, who was in a nursing home, they mutually decided that selling the farm was the best decision for the family.

A good family friend, Fritz, came to David's hospital room and talked to him about the various options he had with selling the cattle. Fritz thought that Great Northern would do an excellent job at auctioning off the cattle. David agreed and wanted Fritz to use his contacts and set up the cattle auction as soon as possible.

I hated hearing about the cattle sale and knew this was a difficult decision for David. It meant he was accepting the fact that he might never be able to farm again, and farming had been his passion since he was a teenager.

Despite the turmoil that David and I were going through on a daily basis, my pregnancy was progressing normally, and for that, I was extremely thankful. The baby continued to move around, especially at night. I found it difficult to sleep comfortably, but I refused to complain, because I knew David was enduring a lot more than I was. I wanted to be able to share more of my pregnancy experiences with my husband, but I felt his illness was taking center stage. My pregnancy was on the back burner. I didn't mind; I would just have liked David to feel the baby kick. There was very little privacy in a hospital room, so I tended to shy away from too much physical contact. I did give David kisses and hugs each evening before I left the hospital to go home.

I missed the close physical contact we once had between us. It was impossible for me to climb into David's hospital bed and be alongside him because I had the extra baby weight. I often sat in whatever chair I found in his room that provided the most comfort for me. We had very little alone time since there were doctors and nurses coming in at all times of the day and night. David was sleeping more and more, and we didn't talk about things as much as we used to. I think David was afraid to talk about death and the reality that he may not be around to see his daughter being born.

Chapter 45

Preparations for the Baby

In between hospital visits and doctor appointments of my own, I tried to prepare the nursery and get ready for the baby who would arrive in two months. During Thanksgiving weekend, my parents helped me pick up a crib from Shopko. I still wanted to get a changing table and a better quality crib mattress. I wasn't sure when I'd get to do this, but if all else failed, I could order some things online or from one of the department stores.

David's health continued to deteriorate during the next several days. He was so swollen that it was almost impossible for him to urinate on his own. One of the nurses put in a Foley catheter so that David's body could release urine into a bag when necessary. At first, David was okay with this, but then after a while, he forgot he had a catheter and asked me to get his portable urinal so he could go to the bathroom.

David was becoming more disorientated, uncomfortable, and anxious. I had the feeling that he somehow sensed his time left on earth was limited. I'm not sure how he felt about this, as we never really discussed it. I know at one point he said that I would need to "take care of things." David had always taken care of the finances and had done much of the calling when it came to repairs on the house. He took on the role of provider at all times. Now I would have to assume most of the responsibilities, and I wasn't sure I knew how!

Chapter 46

Final Chemotherapy Treatment

On Monday, December 13, I was in the room when Dr. K came in to do his rounds. He explained that David's liver functions were up again, almost where they were two weeks ago when chemotherapy started. Dr. K also explained that he could try another round of chemotherapy, but there was only a ten percent chance the treatment would help. David, being the brave and kindhearted man he was, looked at Dr. K and said, "I have a lot to live for!"

So the nurse on duty started another round of chemotherapy drugs. David seemed more anxious and uncomfortable than usual. But in my heart, I knew he was willing to go through anything if it meant he had more time to spend with the baby and me. David was also very confused from the antianxiety drugs. He mumbled things when he was half-asleep most of the day, but I could sense he was relieved to know I was there to hold his hand. I tried to comfort him the best I could.

Chapter 47

Saying Our Good-Byes

On December 14, I woke up early because I had to go to the bathroom. I also wanted to get to the hospital early for my daily visit with David. Just before 8:00 a.m., the phone rang. My sister-in-law, Joanne, asked me to come to the hospital as soon as possible. I could sense by the tone of her voice that something was wrong. What situation would I encounter this time? Would David still be alive when I arrived? I hurried to the hospital as fast as I dared, considering it was winter and I was seven and a half months pregnant. I could only waddle, much less run.

When I arrived at the hospital, Joanne and Pastor Jenny greeted me as I entered David's room. Joanne said we didn't have much time left with David. She and I sat with tears in our eyes, willing them not to fall. I was in a daze and functioning through pure willpower and determination. I sat thinking that this was it; I must face reality. David was going to die. It may be within the hour, or it may be within the next several hours. Somehow, calm washed over me. I think I realized that this was David's time to go and that no matter what I did or how I felt, it was going to happen. I felt God holding my hand and telling me, "Kathy, it is time for David to go. It will be okay. I am with you, and I will help you through this."

Stephanie, the oncology nurse, came in and talked with us. She asked if I wanted David's medicines stopped and the tubes disconnected. I asked her to unhook everything except the morphine. I somehow sensed that David didn't need any of the medications, but I hoped the morphine would take the edge off his pain.

The entire day was a blur of mixed memories and emotions. I remember Joanne calling Brian, one of David's closest friends, and telling him that David wasn't doing well and that he should come to the hospital. Brian came from work and immediately broke down. Brian was an emotional guy, and he hated seeing his friend of many years lying in that hospital bed dying of cancer.

Brian asked if there was anything he could do. I asked him to call my parents, and also Randy and Lynn, other friends of ours. I wanted the family and David's friends to see him one last time to be able to say their good-byes.

Joanne and I went to lunch about 11:30. Neither one of us had much of an appetite, but I knew I had to eat to provide nourishment for our baby and to keep up my strength. Joanne and I said very little to each other. I ate and she moved food slowly around her plate. It had already been an exhausting day for the both of us. We had no idea how long David would live and decided to stay at the hospital.

After lunch, our friend Deb came in to say good-bye to David. She looked at me with heartfelt sympathy but just didn't know what to say. I could understand this sentiment. What does one say to a pregnant woman who is losing her spouse?

A short time later, Randy and Lynn came to say their good-byes. Randy stood by David's bedside and said, "I'll sure miss you, buddy. We had a lot of good times together."

Lynn held David's hand. I could see her holding back the tears, and she appeared distressed. Later on, I found out that while Lynn was in college, she had lost her father to colon cancer. I am sure this visit with David brought back sad memories for her as well.

How one day can drag on is beyond me. The minutes and hours seemed to tick by so slowly that I thought this day would never end! David appeared very anxious. Joanne and I kept reassuring him that everything would be okay. The farm and the cattle were fine.

At one point, I remember telling David that it was okay to let go now. There was no need to fight the pain anymore. The baby and I would be all right. Somehow, I believed he heard me, even in his state of semiconsciousness.

Around 3:30 p.m., my parents, Mark, and Michele arrived from Merrill. My dad looked somber and grim. My mom does not do well in these kinds of situations, and she started to cry as soon as she walked into the room. My parents thought the world of David. They didn't want to see him suffer anymore, but at the same time, they didn't want to lose the son-in-law they had gotten to know and love during the last three years.

It felt good to have my family around for support. I felt wrapped in their love during this horrific time when I needed them the most. My brother Erik showed up a short while later.

Just prior to 4:00 p.m., Stephanie, the head oncology nurse, came in to say her good-byes. She sat by David's bedside and gave a very eloquent speech telling him how much she would miss him and that he was a kindhearted and wonderful man who no longer would have to suffer the pain of cancer.

I cried so many times that day. I felt emotionally drained and physically worn out, but I knew I would be at the hospital until David passed away. I didn't want him to die alone in his hospital room. I wanted him to know that I took our marriage vows seriously, and I would be there "till death do us part."

Joanne's husband, Tom, arrived around 6:00 p.m. He had driven six hours from Indianapolis, Indiana, and made it to the hospital safely. Joanne had kept her emotions in check all day, but when Tom arrived, she broke down and sobbed. She left the room with Tom by her side. I was glad he was there to offer her support. Frankly, I was holding on by a thread and felt that I could only be strong enough to support the baby and myself.

Chapter 48

One Long Night

M y brothers were concerned that I was neglecting my health and suggested that they get some food and bring it in for us to eat. I agreed, because once again, I knew I had to keep up my strength and provide for the baby. But in reality, I wasn't hungry at all.

The hospital staff was very accommodating to my family's needs and allowed us to eat supper in the family lounge. All day long, the hospital staff had provided hospice care for David and offered me anything I could possibly need. I was grateful for their care and concern. At the same time, I just wanted to be alone to spend what remaining time I had with David in peace and quiet without the machines, the medicines, and the gadgets that would no longer help him recover from the cancer that had destroyed his body.

My brother so graciously went to my house to get my glasses, because I knew it could be an extremely long evening. I removed my contacts and gratefully accepted my glasses. I told my parents, Mark, and Michele that they could stay at our house for the night. They said their good-byes to David and left around 8:00 p.m.

Joanne and I settled in for the night. We asked the nurse to give David another dose of antianxiety medication, because he seemed overly restless and anxious. He probably sensed that death wasn't too far off. I'm pretty sure David feared leaving the earthly world behind and those he loved.

Around 10:00 p.m. Joanne and I tried to get some sleep. The chair I was laying in was extremely uncomfortable, especially since I was pregnant and sleeping these days was uncomfortable most of the time anyway. Around 12:30 a.m., David drifted into a semirelaxed sleep, and Joanne went to the family lounge to get some sleep. I tried to fall asleep in the recliner but was unsuccessful.

At 1:30 a.m., I heard David moaning, but he appeared to be resting okay, so I went into the family lounge to rest for a little while. I awoke at 2:45 a.m. to go to the bathroom. Somehow, I sensed that I needed to return to David's room. When I got into the room, David's breathing was very shallow. I was scared and relieved at the same time. I stepped into the hallway and asked a nurse to get Joanne from the family lounge.

Chapter 49

Pain and Sorrow

B y the time Joanne arrived, David had passed away. Joanne called the nurse back into the room, and she confirmed that David had indeed died. This had been one of the longest, most memorable days of my life.

It was now almost 3:00 a.m., and we were instructed to clean out David's room and take his belongings home. The staff needed to clean the room for the next patient. This was the very last thing I wanted to do! Why couldn't this wait until later in the morning? I had just lost my husband and now they were telling me to gather up his things and move on as if it's no big deal!

In a fog of pain and sorrow, Joanne and I gathered David's possessions and put them in a duffel bag that had followed us around the hospital for the last several weeks. The nurses had given David a small, fake Christmas tree that decorated his room. I would most likely be using this as my tree, as I did not intend to put up another tree that Christmas.

When I arrived home, my parents were awake and concerned. I could tell they didn't know what to say. I told them that I was tired and was going to sleep. It had been an extremely long and exhausting day, and I just wanted to try to rest. Unfortunately, at about 7:30 that morning, I woke to the aroma of breakfast cooking in the kitchen. I knew that I wouldn't be able to sleep anymore that day, so I got up and made my way downstairs.

My parents, brother, and sister-in-law were already downstairs, and they asked me why I was awake so early. I told them that I had slept at the hospital the night before. I wasn't ready to face the scrutiny that my family and friends were about to place on me. In my heart, I knew everyone was concerned for my well-being, but my head was screaming, "Just leave me alone. I'll be okay!"

I felt comfort from my family, but I also needed time alone to deal with my grief in my own way. I tried to keep my emotions in check so no one would hover over me. I am an independent person and like having my own space. But in the days to come, I found comfort and security from my family and friends.

Chapter 50

The Funeral

That Thursday, we went to a funeral home to make the arrangements, which was one of the hardest things I had ever done. Before we left for the funeral home, I had selected an outfit that David would wear. It was what he had worn to church just before Christmas, and I knew he would be pleased with my choice. I paired the khaki pants and navy sport coat with a white shirt and Christmas tie.

The funeral director was so good at comforting us. He helped make all the necessary preparations. I felt overwhelmed and saddened that I even had to do this at all. Thankfully, Joanne wrote the obituary, because my writing skills would have failed me miserably at this time. The hymns I chose were ones that David had enjoyed singing on occasion at church. I was grateful that a family friend would sing them at the service.

December 19 should have been a day to celebrate David's birthday. Instead, we held a visitation at our church. I was overwhelmed by the amount of friends and family who came to pay their respects. There were so many times during the visitation that I cried. After a while, I felt like I didn't have any more tears left to shed.

David's funeral was on a blustery, cold day. Pastor Jenny's meditation service was comforting. She spoke about how cancer had chosen to take David's life. God was weeping with us at this time of pain and sorrow.

Chapter 51

Trying to Cope

T he first few weeks following David's death I did everything in my power to stay busy. I didn't want to have time to think. If I had too much time on my hands, I wallowed in self-pity and questioned why God had done this to me. I was angry and disappointed in God.

Those first few weeks I went shopping, bought furniture for the nursery, and continued with my doctor's appointments. I truly think that being pregnant saved me from having a nervous breakdown. I had to stay strong for my baby and myself. There were times, especially late at night when I would lie in bed and cry myself to sleep. I was so lonely and the house felt too quiet and too big for me.

A few days after David's funeral, we prepared the cattle to travel to Fond du Lac to be sold at an auction. Stepping into the barn, I expected David to walk around the corner and greet me with a smile. But I knew this wasn't going to happen. It hurt to look at the handwritten signs that David had posted above the stalls of the uncooperative cows or those cows that had special milking needs.

I continued to keep myself as busy as possible so I wouldn't think too much about being alone. My friends were there when I needed them the most. Brian and Randy assembled the crib. I eagerly began decorating the nursery and preparing myself for the birth of our daughter. Yes, I still considered David to be with me, if not in body then certainly in spirit.

The first month after David passed away, I walked through the quiet, empty house hoping he would come back. I knew that wasn't going to happen, but my heart ached for the one person who truly knew me and had comforted me so many times. I longed for David's embrace and gentle voice telling me that everything would be all right.

I was definitely looking forward to my daughter's birth; however, I didn't recall signing up for the young widow and single mother role. Would I be able to handle the responsibilities of raising our daughter on my own? All I knew is that I would do my best and ask God for his help along the way.

Chapter 52

Baby on the Way

As my due date approached, I went in for a routine prenatal exam. I was told that I could have an elective induction on February 9, 2005. However, on the evening of February 9, I received a call from one of the nurses on the maternity ward. She told me there were too many women in labor at this time, and I wouldn't be having my induction that night. I was extremely disappointed, but again I felt that I had little control over my life.

Early Friday morning on February 11, I woke up at around three o'clock in the morning. I started to feel what I believed were contractions. At 6:00 a.m., I called my sister-in-law, Joanne, and asked her to take me to the hospital. Once settled into a hospital room, the nurse started me on Pitocin to get my contractions into a regular pattern. However, when my gynecologist came to examine me, he informed me that I wasn't in active labor and suggested I go home and wait for labor to start naturally.

I was fed up with doctors giving me advice and directions in general, but I calmly thought through my situation. When my doctor returned an hour later, I asked that he proceed with my induction that day. He warned me that the labor might be long and tiresome. I assured him that I would take whatever came my way and would not blame him for my decision. David and I had waited years to be parents, and I was more than ready to start the next chapter of my life with my daughter.

So before the doctor left, he inserted some medicine into my uterus that started the contractions and began my labor. For the first thirty minutes, I was required to lie in bed and let the medicine take effect. After the initial thirty minutes were up, I walked the hallways of the maternity ward with my birth coach and sister-in-law.

During this time, I wasn't allowed to eat any solid food, so my lunch consisted of popsicles and clear broth—not much to keep my energy level up. By three o'clock that afternoon, I was tired and anxious. When the nurse came in to do an exam at 3:30 p.m., I felt a gush of water on the bed sheets. My water had finally broken! Now I would surely make more progress!

This was a short-lived victory, because I began to feel some major contractions. I cringed and tried to remember to breathe through the pain. Yeah, right! I knew I wouldn't be able to endure hours of this kind of pain, so I asked for an epidural. The anesthesiologist came in around 5:30 p.m. and inserted an epidural that gave me relief from the contractions.

For the next several hours, Joanne and I passed the time watching television, learning to use my new digital camera, and trying to guess what time my daughter would be born. Finally, around 10:00 p.m., the nurse informed me that I was fully dilated and to start pushing. I was hesitant with the first few pushes, but for the next two hours, I pushed as I had never pushed before. This was the hardest thing that I had to endure, well, the second hardest thing. The first was watching my husband slowly die from cancer.

The nurse announced that my daughter's head was stuck in the birth canal. Great! After all this work, I thought I'd have to go in for an emergency C-section. I didn't want to set foot in an operating room! The pain and suffering David endured during the last two months was still a clear memory. I kept hoping that a C-section wouldn't be necessary.

Chapter 53

Anna Is Here

T he doctor on call that evening suggested a vacuum to help ease my daughter out of the birth canal. He assured me this procedure wouldn't harm my daughter and would help me deliver her with few complications. I was hesitant, but truthfully, I just wanted to see my daughter and hear her first cry! I agreed to allow the doctor to perform the vacuum method.

Thankfully, the procedure went well. After positioning the little suction cup on Anna's head, the doctor used a gentle vacuum and after three more pushes, I finally heard my newborn daughter's cry! Anna Davida Depping was born at 1:15 a.m. on February 12, 2005. She weighed nine pounds and was twenty-one inches long!

I started crying the moment they placed Anna on my tummy! This was such a bittersweet moment for me. I was overjoyed to have the daughter I had longed for, but at the same time, I longed for David to be with me to share in the joy. Unfortunately, I started hemorrhaging, but the doctor massaged my uterus and the bleeding stopped. After I was stitched up and Anna was put into warm clothes and a blanket, we had some anxious visitors. My parents and David's mom, as well as Joanne, came in to admire our small miracle. Anna brought us all so much joy after losing David just two months earlier.

The next two days, I bonded with my daughter in the hospital. I needed time to heal and prepare myself for the duties of being a single mom. Anna was a very content baby and bonded with me while I nursed her.

Chapter 54

Single Mom Woes

The first month after Anna's birth, I struggled with being a new mom and suffered serious sleep deprivation. One evening as I tried to console Anna, I looked up to heaven and asked God to help me out—I couldn't take much more! I had a good cry and Anna finally fell asleep. There were several moments like this during the first few months of Anna's life, but somehow we made it through together.

Our house felt too big and held too many memories. I longed for the companionship and love that David brought into my life. I believe these first several months were my survival period. I went through the routines and daily tasks because I had to. I wanted to be a good mother to Anna. Some days she was my sole motivation to get up and continue my day. I was moving on the best I knew how.

Anna was an extremely good baby. However, she really liked to eat! So every two to three hours I was awake feeding her. I noticed my eyes looked tired from lack of sleep. I had always had lazy eyes, but they were worse now than before. There was no way I could wear my contacts, and my tiredness showed even when I wore my glasses!

Chapter 55

Life Changes and Moving On

When Anna turned six months old, I consulted an eye specialist. She tried to fit me with a stronger prescription, but that did very little to correct my eye problems. So in August of 2005, I underwent eye muscle surgery. After the operation, my eyes were so red and sore I looked as if I had a terrible hangover! But within about a month after surgery, I noticed my eyes were working better together, and they weren't crossing at all. I was pleased with the results and anxious to begin wearing my contacts again.

I began to feel a little restless and wanted to get back into the working world, at least on a part-time basis. So when Anna was ten months old, I began to substitute teach again. It felt good to get out of the house and interact with adults in the teaching field.

In the summer of 2005, my parents moved near us in Howards Grove. They had planned to move to our area earlier when David got sick. They wanted to be closer to Anna and me and help when I needed them. I have to admit that during the summer and autumn of 2005, I really appreciated their help, especially when they cared for Anna.

The new year brought many changes for my small family. In February, Anna turned a year old, and we had a birthday celebration with the immediate family.

Shortly after Anna's first birthday, we were invited to a birthday party for Stephanie's son. I had not been out socially in a long time, and Anna and I both enjoyed the party very much.

As we were leaving, I met one of Nick's, Stephanie's husband's, friends in passing. It was a very quick introduction, because Anna and I were headed out the door.

During a telephone conversation with Stephanie sometime later, we happened on the subject of dating. She asked me if I was ready to start dating again. I thought about it a few minutes, and then I replied, after a few minutes of thinking about it, that I was. Stephanie, the concerned and kind friend that she is, gave her husband's friend Brett my telephone number.

Chapter 56

Meeting Someone New

I was pleasantly surprised when Brett called me the next day! He and I talked for two hours and got to know each other. When Brett called again the next evening, I sucked up every ounce of courage I had and asked him if he wanted to go out on a date. Somehow, I found the confidence to do something that I normally would never have done. I think Brett was a little taken aback, but he accepted my invitation.

The evening of our first date, I took Anna to my parents to spend the night. I wanted to get ready for the date without having to watch my active toddler, and I needed to get my nerves under control. It had been six years since I had dated, and I was stepping into the dating scene with a young daughter to think about as well. I was looking for someone who liked children and would treat my daughter with kindness, and at the same time, treat me as if I was important as well.

Brett arrived and we went out on a dinner date. The conservation flowed smoothly. I was quite surprised by how much we had in common. We really enjoyed each other's company. After dinner, I invited Brett to my house. We continued our conversation over drinks and soft background music. It got late and Brett decided it was time to go home. Before he left, he asked if we could see each other again.

I was hesitant to introduce Anna to someone I had just met, but at the same time, I didn't want to rely on my parents to watch Anna whenever I went out. I strived to be a good mom, while at the same time, learning how to have a social life. I didn't want Anna to be attached to a guy if he and I weren't going to be in a serious relationship.

The following weekend Brett came over for supper. At first, Anna was shy and reluctant to get too close to him. After all, she had me all to herself most of the time, and she wasn't too willing to share me with someone else. After a little while, she warmed up to Brett, and by the time Anna went to bed, she had made a new friend.

Chapter 57

Moving and Dating Again

B rett and I began dating. We enjoyed going out with each other and having adult time. It had been a long while since I was able to enjoy myself with other adults. Brett also spent time with Anna and me at home. He did a great job of including her in many of our outings. Sometimes we would go to his parents' house. Anna loved it when Brett's nieces entertained her. Other times, we would spend a quiet evening at home watching a movie or just relaxing.

In April 2006, Anna and I moved into a house in the city of Plymouth. I really liked our new home. It was close to the city park and a pool. Once Anna started school, she would be able to walk to the nearest elementary just a few blocks from our house.

Brett and I continued dating and spent as much time together as his work schedule would allow. We all have little quirks or things that irritate our significant other. I have to admit that I could get a little obsessive with keeping my house clean.

Brett was a snorer, so it was a struggle for us to sleep together. I'm a light sleeper and certain noises keep me awake. I really wanted this relationship to work, as I deeply cared for Brett. I think we both lost a lot of sleep, because we both worried about each other!

Chapter 58

Single Once Again

As Christmas 2006 approached, I was feeling exhausted and disappointed. Some of my feelings were tied to my new job that required me to get up early each morning. I was fed up with trying to juggle a full-time job and being a full-time parent. So I decided to give up the job and concentrate on being a good mother to Anna.

Around this time, I also sensed a change in my relationship with Brett. Neither one of us wanted to admit it, but things weren't working out. I couldn't sleep well because Brett's snoring kept me awake. At the same time, he slept restlessly because he was afraid he was keeping me awake. We felt like we were in a no-win situation.

Christmas came and went. Brett and I didn't want to ruin each other's holiday by talking about our relationship. By the end of December, I could feel Brett starting to pull away from me a little at a time. We mutually decided things weren't working out for us and that we should go our separate ways. Fortunately, Brett and I remain friends, and I credit him with giving me the chance to pick up my life and start dating again. I certainly hope that one day he finds someone to share his life with as well.

New Year's Eve 2006 was another turning point in my life. I was single once again and really hated the thought of being alone. I wished for someone special to share my life with again. My daughter meant everything to me, but I wanted adult companionship in my life.

As the new year approached, I reflected on my life. I didn't want to go to bars to socialize and meet people. So I took a chance with an Internet dating service once again. A year earlier, I had established an account with Match.com. I updated my profile with this site and hoped for the best.

Chapter 59

Internet Dating

The first few weeks I looked at the website faithfully. To my disappointment, most of the guys were either older than I was or lived too far away. I didn't want a long-distance relationship with someone. My first priority was taking care of my daughter.

I decided to broaden my horizons and added my profile to Yahoo! Personals. Again, I wasn't putting too much faith in the site but thought I might as well try it. To my surprise, the next day, I received an e-mail from a single guy from Sheboygan Falls. Well, at least it was close to Plymouth. He said he knew me from church. Quickly, I began paging through the church directory to find a picture of this guy. Even after seeing his picture, I didn't recognize him at all! How could it be that we had been going to the same church for a number of years and I had no idea who he was?

After careful consideration, I decided to respond to Ryan's e-mail. I wrote about things I like to do and the type of music I enjoy. Surprisingly, we had a lot in common. We both liked eighties music, the outdoors, and children.

Ryan and I continued sending e-mails to each other for several days. I was hoping we could have a verbal conversation, so I sent Ryan my home phone number. I was pleasantly surprised when Ryan called that evening after I had put Anna to bed.

We talked about our various interests. The conversation flowed so smoothly that we spoke for several hours that evening. The next night Ryan called again. We talked on the phone for hours! As we wrapped up our call, Ryan asked me if I would like to go out to dinner sometime. I agreed, and we planned on a Wednesday dinner date.

Chapter 60

Dating Ryan

That date was one I won't forget. I was like a nervous teenage girl going out for the first time! I think I changed clothes about five times. By the time the doorbell rang, I had pulled myself together enough to notice this handsome guy standing at my door. He was dressed in a light blue sweater and jeans. Did I happen to tell him my favorite color was blue? I also noticed his bright blue eyes and warm smile. Ryan was at least six feet tall and had a larger build than most of the other guys I had previously dated.

Our drive to the restaurant was filled with conversation. We sure didn't run out of things to talk about. We had more in common than I thought. Once we ordered dinner, we continued to converse. I felt completely at ease with Ryan.

I don't think either one of us wanted our date to end, so I asked him in for a nightcap. I lit a fire in the hearth and we continued talking. We both realized the time was approaching midnight, and we had to get up for work in the morning! We reluctantly said our good-byes for the evening.

The next day I was exhausted, but giddy and content. For the first time in months, I felt like someone really liked me! Ryan seemed like a genuinely nice guy, and I enjoyed his company very much. For the next several days, we talked on the phone.

The following Friday, Ryan and I were again talking on the telephone. I was already in my pajamas and wanted to go to sleep, but he persuaded me to let him come over, even though it was already eleven o'clock.

Chapter 61

Another Snorer

As he drifted off to sleep, I began to hear Ryan snore. *No* way! Did I just gravitate toward guys who snored? The next day, I mentioned my fears to Ryan. I had broken off one relationship because that person had a snoring problem. I wasn't going to get seriously involved with another guy who snored. He needed to do something to alleviate his snoring. I didn't want to build a relationship with Ryan and feel exhausted all the time.

One evening, Ryan came over with a gadget that he said was supposed to wake him up when he started snoring. The apparatus, which he wore on his wrist, was supposed to shock him awake when he started snoring. Unfortunately, the device didn't work, and we were back to square one. What was the next possible solution to the snoring problem?

After some sleepless nights for both of us, Ryan gave in and made an appointment with an ear, nose, and throat specialist. The doctor told Ryan his tonsils were large, and his tongue rolled back in his throat when he fell asleep. The doctor also suggested that Ryan take a sleep study to see if he had sleep apnea.

The tests concluded that Ryan had sleep apnea. He would stop breathing several times each night! I was shocked and frightened to learn that this happens, and that it can take a toll on a person's heart.

Chapter 62

Ryan Moves In

On April 17, 2007, Ryan was fitted with a CPAP (continuous positive airway pressure) machine. This machine would be a lifesaver. It would allow Ryan to breathe better at night, and allow us to sleep in the same bed without causing me to lose unnecessary sleep.

Ryan and I also started talking about marriage in the spring of 2007. I really didn't want a big wedding. I didn't need a big wedding to show Ryan how much I loved and cared about him. I would be satisfied with a small, simple ceremony. However, this being Ryan's first marriage, he wanted a big wedding. I went along with his ideas, because I realized it was unfair of me to have him give up his one chance at having a large wedding celebration.

In early May 2007, Anna had vents put in her ears. It had taken me six months to convince our doctor that she had ear problems and needed to see a specialist. The ear, nose, and throat doctor looked in her ears and recommended that she would benefit from ear vents. As most parents know, surgery for their child can be a little scary, especially since you have no control over what is being done!

But Anna came out of surgery (minus her adenoids) and recovered very well. For the next few days, Anna's ears drained a pink-tinged liquid, but I learned this was a normal reaction.

I was so grateful to have Ryan with us during that time. He stayed overnight the day Anna came home from surgery. He claimed he wanted to help me with her. Whatever the reason, I grew accustomed to Ryan coming to my house each evening after work. It was wonderful having a male role model in the house again!

Chapter 63

Getting Remarried

Ryan proposed to me on June 18, 2007. Granted, it wasn't a unique or romantic proposal, but it came from the heart, and that's all that really mattered. I was happy to have found someone who loved me and treated my daughter like his own. We chose April 12, 2008, as the date for our upcoming wedding.

Those who know me well know I like to be organized, so wedding preparations began shortly after we became engaged. I booked the church, the reception hall, and the photographer all within a few days after Ryan's proposal.

Wedding preparations were moving along smoothly; however, I couldn't help but feel guilty for moving on with my life. Somehow, I felt like I was betraying David's memory. Realistically, I knew David would want me to be happy and move on with my life. I'd have to work on sorting out these feelings during the next several months while Ryan and I prepared for our wedding.

During the summer of 2007, Anna reached certain milestones as well. She began using the potty chair more frequently. She also started refusing to take naps. One afternoon in early September, I spent three hours trying to get her down for a nap. Unfortunately, she only slept an hour that day. When Anna napped, I could relax or regroup and get things done.

We received disappointing news at the end of September; our ministers announced they would be leaving our church after twenty years of service. Ryan and I were upset. We had been looking forward to having Pastor Jenny and Pastor Jim marry us. We prayed there would be an interim minister in place before our wedding in April.

Chapter 64

Dealing with Major Life Changes

In October, I began to think about seeing a counselor again. I had started counseling when Anna was a toddler. I credit my therapist with helping me work through some emotionally difficult times in my life. There were certain events and dates that triggered the pain and grief of losing David. I chose to stop counseling sessions when I first started dating again, but now I felt a need to talk through my doubts and concerns with my previous counselor.

During the third week of October 2007, Ryan and I took a vacation to Las Vegas. This was the first time I had been away from Anna for an extended period. I enjoyed our vacation, but at the same time, I missed Anna terribly. My allergies were bothering me, and I truly felt by being away from my daughter, a little piece of me was missing. I have to admit it was good to get away, and I returned refreshed and ready to be a better mom to my daughter.

In December 2007, I received some startling news about David's uncle Elmer. He had just been diagnosed with colon cancer. I thought this was an ironic time for his diagnosis, as it was almost three years since David had passed away from the same type of cancer. Fortunately, Elmer's cancer was diagnosed early, and he is still with us today!

The winter of 2007–2008 was a difficult one for Anna. She suffered from several ear infections and seemed to be on antibiotics continually. I felt so bad for her each time we had to go to the doctor's office for treatment. I was concerned that the constant ear infections might affect her hearing.

Anna had her three-year-old screening with the Plymouth School District at the end of January. When they tested her hearing the first time, she didn't do well, but I was amazed at how well she tested in the verbal and social areas.

Fortunately, two months later when she was retested, her hearing was normal. I breathed a huge sigh of relief!

Chapter 65

Our Wedding

Our wedding day on April 12, 2008, was cold, wet, and gloomy. Not the kind of weather I had hoped for when we were planning this special day more than a year ago. Since you can't change the weather, I decided to make the best of it no matter what! Ryan and I had an intimate wedding ceremony and enjoyed our reception as well. I was marrying a man who loved me unconditionally and was willing to be a stepfather for my little girl.

Chapter 66

Anna's Glasses

At the end of April 2008, Anna had her first eye screening. Our eye doctor noticed her right eye tended to cross inward. I cringed and thought I had given my daughter my eye problems. We scheduled an appointment with a pediatric ophthalmologist. She suggested Anna be fitted with glasses to correct her vision problems before starting 4K in the fall.

I let Anna choose the color and style of glass frames she wanted. She selected the cutest little purple frames, and I was pleased at how well the glasses looked on her. Anna was the proudest little girl I knew sporting her new glasses to anyone who cared to notice!

Chapter 67

My Health Scare

The first week of June 2008, I went to my gynecologist for a routine annual exam. During the exam, my doctor found what he believed was a lump on my left breast and suggested I get a mammogram as soon as possible. My initial reaction was how the heck could God do this to me again! Cancer, no way! I didn't want to leave my daughter without a mother too. Surely, God didn't want that to happen. I kept thinking the worst, but I hoped for the best possible outcome.

Fortunately, the mammogram showed normal breast tissue. Whatever my doctor had felt was just lumpy breast tissue. I was so relieved and thanked God for helping me through this scare.

Chapter 68

Adding to Our Family

Ryan and I had talked about having another child as soon as possible. However, after several months of trying to conceive the natural way, nothing happened. At first, I didn't want to consider going through fertility treatments again. I clearly remembered how challenging it was both physically and emotionally. But as the summer months wore on, I began to reconsider. After all, I had been through fertility treatments before and had some idea of what to expect. Ryan and I decided to wait until the end of August before making an appointment with a fertility specialist.

Chapter 69

More Fertility Treatments

I
n early September 2008, Ryan and I went for a consultation with a fertility specialist. It was reassuring to hear that the doctor thought I could get pregnant again. However, I was forty years old now, and it might be a little more difficult than when I got pregnant with Anna at thirty-five.

I was willing to go through the hormone shots and repeated examinations if it meant I would get pregnant with another child. In the back of my mind, I kept thinking that this would be my last opportunity to have another child. I wanted Ryan to be able to go through a pregnancy with me and have his own biological child. Ryan was such a great father figure for Anna, and another child would add more energy and happiness to our family.

After a battery of tests, the doctor found my FSH (follicle-stimulating hormone) levels high. So after my next monthly cycle, he put me on birth control pills that I hoped would lower my FSH levels. Ideally, the doctor wanted to see a FSH level of twelve or below before he proceeded with the next step in an IVF procedure.

Chapter 70

Another IVF Journey

During November and December 2008, I dutifully took a birth control pill each day. However, it was a rough early winter for Anna. Just before Thanksgiving, she developed an ear infection. Unfortunately, the antibiotics she was taking didn't help, and we ended up in an emergency room on Thanksgiving Day with a very sick little girl! My poor baby had pus and gunk draining out of her ear and down her cheek. As a mother, I just wanted her to feel better as fast as humanly possible!

As Christmas approached, I began feeling depressed and a little forlorn. December 15, the anniversary of David's death, triggered memories that I have tried very hard to put on the back burner. I attended a service of remembrance at our church that helped me put things into perspective, and I was able to enjoy the holiday season.

At the end of December, Ryan and I went to our fertility specialist for injection training. I needed a refresher course, and Ryan needed to learn what medicines I would take and where the injections would go. I wasn't looking forward to beginning these shots again. I had clear memories of the painful injection site from my previous IVF cycle in 2004.

At the beginning of January 2009, I started taking Follistim and Repronex shots. The Follistim pen in my upper thigh was no big deal, because I felt very little or no pain. Occasionally, I would poke myself too hard with the small needles and end up with a bruise on my upper thigh or leg.

During each IVF cycle, I was monitored very closely to determine where my hormone levels were and how my ovaries were being stimulated.

The goal is for the ovaries to produce multiple eggs so they can be collected and fertilized with Ryan's sperm.

This seems like a simple process, right? Well, I have definitely oversimplified the procedure and tried to make it easier to understand, because not everyone has had to go through fertility treatments.

I kept going in for ultrasounds to determine how many eggs were maturing. As the hormone injections continued, I began to feel like a human pincushion. My thighs were bruised and very tender to the touch. I was hopeful that by the beginning of February I would be pregnant.

On January 22, 2009, I had the egg retrieval done. It went well, and the doctor was able to gather four mature eggs to fertilize with Ryan's sperm. I was encouraged; this was the number I had when I became pregnant with Anna!

On January 28, 2009, the embryos were implanted. The doctor felt two were good quality. Then for the next three days, I was on complete bed rest. As I have mentioned before, I am not one to sit around and do nothing, so for me this is the hardest part of the cycle. However, this time around, I had an extremely sore back and my butt hurt from sitting in one place for so long. I kept telling myself that this would be worth it if I became pregnant.

During this time, Anna began to act up. She knew something was going on and wanted her mommy to do things with her. After my three days of bed rest, I was more than willing to spend quality time with my daughter.

The next step in the IVF journey was to wait ten days for a pregnancy test. For someone with little patience, this was very difficult for me.

Chapter 71

Tough Decisions

On February 6, 2009, a nurse called with the results of my pregnancy test. The result was positive; however, my hormone levels weren't quite as high as they would have liked them to be. The nurse advised me to be cautiously optimistic and return the next Monday for more blood work.

That weekend, I prayed that my hormone levels would increase. I really wanted this pregnancy to work and for us to welcome another child into our family. However, when I went in for my second blood draw, the results were not good. My hormone levels had decreased. I was advised to stop taking all the medicine I was prescribed. Now I had to wait for my monthly cycle to come again. I was extremely disappointed and sad. They always tell you there are no guarantees, but that doesn't make the pain and disappointment hurt any less.

After some careful discussion, Ryan and I decided to make another appointment with the fertility specialist and inquire about our options. Previously, the doctor had briefly mentioned the possibility of doing a cycle of IVF using donor eggs. I was a little skeptical at first, but I truly wanted another child.

On February 12, 2009, Anna celebrated her fourth birthday. On that day, I reflected on the things I was thankful for in my life. I felt thankful for my daughter, who has been fairly healthy. I felt thankful that I was given another chance at love, as I had met Ryan and we married. Ryan has been my support system through many rough times. He continues to love me even when I am hard to live with, and he does things he doesn't really like to do.

Chapter 72

Try, Try Again

During this time, a few of Ryan's friends were asking us when we were going to have another child. I know they meant well, but each time I was asked, I grew a little more defensive and a little angrier with myself. Why wasn't I able to get pregnant like some of our friends? I believed that if they knew how hard we were trying to conceive, they wouldn't be giving us such a hard time. In the meantime, I gritted my teeth and told them we were still trying.

At the end of February, we had another consultation with our fertility specialist. He suggested we use donor eggs in our next attempt at becoming pregnant. Unfortunately, you need to go through several loopholes before starting an IVF cycle.

First, a counselor evaluated us to see if we would make good parents to a child who was not technically our biological child. Second, we had to go through the difficult process of choosing a donor. Let me tell you, looking through paperwork to choose a donor is not easy. But Ryan and I finally agreed on a woman who had donated her eggs before. We wanted to choose a donor who would help us conceive another child.

Some of you may be reading this and thinking why would anyone do this? Maybe it's against your religious beliefs, or maybe you just don't believe this is a good way to have children. I am not saying that IVF is for everyone, but for Ryan and me, this seemed like the best choice. I wasn't able to conceive my own biological child this time. I believed that if I were to get pregnant, this child would still have some of Ryan's genetic makeup.

Believe me when I say that Ryan and I went through many hours of decision making before we decided to invest both financially and emotionally in the IVF journey. We decided we would try one more round of IVF and see what happened. I have always been one to remain optimistic.

At the beginning of March, I pleaded with Ryan to let me get Anna a puppy. He was very reluctant at first, because Anna wasn't comfortable around dogs. I also thought that having a pet would teach Anna some responsibility and respect for animals. So we added a teddy bear puppy to our family the first weekend in March. It took Anna a little while to get used to Brandi, but they soon became inseparable.

On March 14, 2009, we chose a donor, and then we had to wait for our donor to be tested. The next step in the donor IVF cycle was synchronizing my monthly cycle with the donor's monthly cycle. This wasn't as easy as it sounds. First, I had to go on birth control pills once again to regulate my cycle. Next, I had to wait for our donor to get her monthly cycle. In the meantime, our donor was standing up in a wedding in May, so the doctor thought it would be wise to wait until after that time to start our IVF cycle.

Once again, I was at the mercy of another person's schedule. I felt like I had absolutely no control when this next IVF cycle would happen.

The first week of April 2009, we began remodeling our basement. Ryan and I decided it was time to finish off at least half of it. The contractors worked very efficiently, and by April 15, they had an egress window installed. They also worked on all the electrical outlets and drywall. It was an exciting process to see, because I knew we would use the basement much more once it was remodeled.

Chapter 73

Family Health Scare

Toward the end of April, my mother-in-law Christine (Chris) had a health scare.

On a Wednesday evening, she passed out in the kitchen. Luckily, her husband Roy was there and caught her before she fell. When she regained consciousness, she began to vomit blood. Roy called 9-1-1. Ryan's sister called us from the emergency room to explain the situation. At this point, the doctor was examining Chris and trying to figure out why she had vomited blood. Ryan and I didn't sleep very well that evening. We both worried about his mom.

The following morning, I had to be up early to take Brandi to be spayed. Ryan called me and started getting very emotional, which was unlike him. He told me his dad had phoned him after he had stepped away from the hospital for a while. Roy was crying and appeared upset. The doctors were still trying to diagnose what was wrong with Chris. I told Ryan I would call our pastor and ask that she go to the hospital and offer prayers and guidance for the family.

I arrived at the hospital just before 8:00 a.m. Chris was in the ICU. This was an extremely emotional time for me as well. Being back in the ICU triggered some bad memories for me. Fortunately, Chris wasn't in the same room that David had occupied. I still have trouble going to certain floors of the hospital or entering certain room numbers. I was in that hospital for eight consecutive weeks with David, and I didn't want to be there any longer than necessary.

However, I sucked up my courage and went into Chris's room to see how she was doing. She looked extremely pale and seemed exhausted.

Doctors had inserted a tube into her nose and down her throat. It was supposed to remove any blood still left in her stomach. Seeing this didn't bother me too much, as I had a tube in my nose once when I had a bowel obstruction.

Pastor Kathryn arrived shortly. She held Chris's hand and offered prayers and healing. After our pastor left, I tried to let Chris rest, but unfortunately, each time she started to doze off, someone would come to check her vitals or try to draw blood. Chris was so dehydrated it was virtually impossible to draw any blood from her. I felt so bad and wished that I could do something to make her feel better. I am the kind of person who absolutely hates seeing my loved ones in any type of pain. I often wished I could take a magic wand and make the pain go away.

Around 10:45 a.m., I decided to locate my friend, an oncology nurse. She knew many of the doctors, and I wanted her to introduce me to a gastrointestinal specialist. The general doctor told us the bleeding in Chris's stomach was due to an ulcer from prolonged use of Naproxen. I'm not a medical doctor by any means, but that just didn't make sense to me. I believed Chris needed a second opinion from a gastrointestinal specialist, and she needed one quickly!

Fortunately, my friend came to my rescue again. She introduced me to a gastro specialist. I spoke to him about David's previous condition, and then I mentioned that I'd like to have him talk with my mother-in-law. The specialist handed me his business card, and I graciously thanked him for his time.

I took his card to Chris's room, showed it to her, and explained that this doctor specialized in gastrointestinal issues. I suggested that she might want to consult with him and see if they could properly diagnose her symptoms.

The afternoon wore on, and I sat quietly while she tried to rest.

Later, I again suggested to Chris and Roy that maybe they should consult with the gastrointestinal specialist. I could sense Roy was overwhelmed with everything going on around him. I cautiously asked him if he would like me to see if I could set up a consultation with the specialist, and Roy and Chris agreed.

It felt good to do something proactive for my mother-in-law regarding her health. I had dealt with a number of doctors at this hospital when David was ill. If I had learned one thing, it was that you needed to be positive and seek the best medical advice possible. Sometimes that meant seeking the advice of a specialist or getting a second opinion when a diagnosis was questionable.

The next afternoon when I went to visit Chris at the hospital, she seemed a little better. She had talked to the gastrointestinal specialist. After reviewing her chart and discussing her health history, the doctor discovered that air was being trapped in her stomach after continued use of a CPAP machine.

Several years ago, Chris had acid reflux surgery. The previous acid reflux surgery allowed her relief from acid reflux. Air would go down her throat, but would usually not come back up! Therefore, prolonged use of the CPAP machine had caused a build-up of air in her stomach. The buildup of air in her stomach had caused an ulcer which broke off and caused Chris to vomit blood. Consequently, Chris could no longer use the CPAP machine.

I was so glad to hear that the specialist had diagnosed Chris's condition! Now she would be able to recuperate and get the treatment she needed. Sometimes it really pays to be persistent.

Chapter 74

Another Round of IVF

I was growing impatient. I waited anxiously for more information from our fertility doctor regarding when I would be able to begin another IVF cycle. Waiting is such a tiresome task, especially when you're looking forward to a certain outcome. Truthfully, I just wanted to get through the whole process and settle into either being a mom or moving on with life.

Finally, in early June 2009, I started with another IVF cycle. Our donor responded very well to hormone treatments and produced twenty-four eggs! I was amazed and pleasantly surprised. Granted, many of these eggs would be immature or postmature and not used in the fertilization process. But I remained hopeful. As directed by the fertility specialist, I began taking hormone injections again.

This time around, I had two embryos implanted into my uterus. The doctor sounded very hopeful as we left the fertility clinic, and I began another three days of complete bed rest. For some reason, I had terrible leg cramps and my back ached from sitting in one spot for so long, but I was determined to see the process through. I kept telling myself that this would all be worth it if I became pregnant.

Ten days after implantation, I went back for a pregnancy test. When a nurse called and told me I was pregnant, I was overjoyed! It finally worked! I called Ryan right away and told him the good news. We were very selective in who we shared our information with. It was very early in the pregnancy, and I didn't want to have to explain to anyone if something were to happen.

Chapter 75

Pregnancy Complications

The last two to three weeks in July 2009 were very difficult for me. I started spotting and was extremely concerned that I was going to miscarry. Ryan called our fertility doctor who advised us to come in for an early ultrasound. He wanted to determine the development of the embryo. The doctor located the yolk sac, but it was too early to see a heartbeat. I was scared and felt a little let down after that appointment. It would be two more weeks before I was able to see the doctor again.

During the next fourteen days, I was on bed rest. Each time I tried to walk around or do any kind of physical activity, I would start to spot. In my gut, I felt something was terribly wrong with this pregnancy. I felt out of control. I just wanted a definite answer from our fertility specialist.

On August 24, 2009, I went for another ultrasound. As I drove to my appointment, I prayed I was still pregnant and the embryo would continue to develop. The doctor began the ultrasound, but I could tell by the grave look on his face that the news wasn't good. He looked at me and said, "Kathy, I'm afraid that you had a miscarriage."

I was devastated! The doctor instructed me to stop taking all medications and to wait for my next period. The only thing I could think of was getting dressed and getting as far away from the clinic as possible!

When I got to my vehicle, I sat there for several minutes contemplating the news. Now what? I would wait until I was on the highway before I called Ryan. I didn't want to break down and get too upset, because I had an hour's drive home. Once on the highway, I dialed Ryan's cell. He was waiting for my call. He asked how the appointment went, and I told him not well at all. I explained that I had a miscarriage, and the doctor wanted me to stop taking all medications. Ryan sounded disappointed but sympathetic. I wanted nothing more than to be in his arms and hear him tell me everything would be all right.

Ryan and I talked for a little while longer, and then he suggested I drive to the farm. We would talk some more and he'd give me a big hug. At this point, I was crying and trying very hard not to break down during the drive home. I was devastated! How could this happen to me? I was upset, but at the same time a little relieved. Now I could slowly work at moving forward. I needed to decide my next step.

Chapter 76

Dealing with Miscarriage and Loss

During the next several weeks, I found it difficult to talk about the miscarriage. It seemed many of our friends were expecting and that made me jealous and angry. I wanted to be one of those women, but I knew that was no longer a reality for me. I felt like the entire summer had literally passed me by, and I had nothing to show for it.

My body slowly found its natural rhythms. I got my period at the end of August, and it was heavier than normal. I knew then that my body was doing what it was supposed to be doing, but I also felt it betrayed me. Why wasn't I able to get pregnant and stay pregnant?

Unfortunately, I had to return to the fertility clinic once every two weeks so the nurses could monitor my hormone levels. I dreaded each visit to the clinic. I wanted to be as far away from that place as humanly possible. But on August 31, I went in for blood work and found out my HCG (human chorionic gonadotropin) level went down to five hundred and something. I needed continued monitoring until no trace of the pregnancy hormone remained in my system.

Meanwhile, I was excited to see my little girl go off to her first day of four-year-old kindergarten. I admit that I am an overprotective mom, because I was used to being with Anna most of the time. But as Labor Day drew near, I was anxious to see how she would do at school. My daughter is an inquisitive and very bright child, and she did really well adjusting to being in school half days. I was the one who had a hard time adjusting to her being in school. I found myself picking her up early on more than one occasion!

After several trips to the fertility clinic for routine blood work, on October 4, 2009, I finally tested negative for the HCG hormone. It had taken a good six to eight weeks for my body to adjust and get back to a normal level. I was very grateful that I wouldn't have to endure anymore trips to the fertility clinic.

Chapter 77

Adoption as an Option

During this time, Ryan and I started discussing adoption as way to add to our family. I wasn't quite sure how to go about getting information, so I started researching online. There were a number of agencies in Wisconsin, but we weren't sure which ones were reputable. I consulted with a family attorney, and she checked with other attorneys around the state. We chose two Wisconsin agencies and set up informational meetings with each of them.

In late September and early October, Anna battled a terrible cough. I finally took her to an Urgent Care only to discover that she had bronchitis! I felt bad because I had waited to take her to the doctor thinking her symptoms would improve over time. But as the autumn weather got colder, Anna's symptoms got worse.

Finally, I took her to our general practitioner who suggested she use an inhaler. The first time I tried to get Anna to use the device it was a terrible struggle! She was hesitant and fought with me for more than an hour before finally agreeing to use the inhaler. Fortunately, this helped with her symptoms for a little while.

The first informational adoption meeting Ryan and I attended was in early November 2009. I came away feeling overwhelmed and discouraged. Because of my age and previous marriages, we would only qualify to adopt a child from Bulgaria. If we chose the domestic adoption route, we would have to be put on a wait list. After some discussion, Ryan and I chose to be placed on the wait list for a domestic adoption.

Ryan and I decided to explore another adoption agency and compare options. When I spoke with someone on the phone from the other agency, I was pleasantly surprised. This agency offered a lottery process. In December and again in May, the agency would hold a drawing and chose names. If your name was chosen, you would be eligible for the adoption program. I thought our chances with the second agency were a little better. Who knew how long we would have to wait to be chosen by the first agency? Personally, I have never been lucky and have not won anything in a lottery before, but maybe this time my luck would change.

Chapter 78

Starting Our Adoption Journey

O ne day in early May, the telephone rang. One of the social workers from the adoption agency was calling to inform us that our name had been chosen from the lottery. I was overjoyed and Ryan was shocked! Now the real work would begin.

The first step was a preliminary interview with our social worker. We discussed what type of program we wanted to be in and the ethnic background of the child we would consider adopting. I had never really thought about an ethnic background of a child. This was never a big issue for Ryan or me. We would love another child no matter what the skin color. However, our social worker brought up a very good point. If our community is predominately Caucasian, a child of African American or even Asian background may feel extremely uncomfortable once they begin to enter their school years.

We decided to proceed with the domestic adoption program and be placed with a Caucasian child or a child from an Asian or Hispanic background. Personally, I wouldn't mind having a child with a different ethnic background than mine. I could embrace the differences and find community members who would be good role models for my adopted child.

After our initial interview, I began to fill out endless amounts of paperwork. Many of the forms were very time consuming and required a lot of thought and explanation. I generally dive in and get tasks completed quickly, but Ryan is quite the opposite. He procrastinates for as long as possible before getting something done, especially if it involves writing or anything thought provoking.

I worked on the paperwork most of the summer of 2010. It kept me busy when I wasn't taking Anna to swim lessons or spending time with her at the park.

There were a few times I got extremely frustrated and wondered why all this hoopla was necessary. Most biological parents don't have to go through this much just to have a child. Why did we?

In August, Ryan and I attended education-training sessions at the Lutheran Social Services office. At first, I was skeptical about how much I would learn. I already knew how to be a parent! I had taken care of Anna for the last five years, and I believe I had done a darn good job of parenting. What more was there to learn?

Chapter 79

Relating to Others about Infertility Problems

Well, I learned there are other couples out there who have suffered through infertility issues like Ryan and I have. In fact, it was somewhat reassuring to know that I wasn't the only person in the world with infertility problems. Sometimes, when you are in the middle of a fertility treatment, it is difficult to see past the immediate future. All I wanted was to be pregnant and have another biological child. I was oblivious to those around me going through the same or similar situation.

During our educational training, I also let go some of the grief I had bottled up inside of me after my miscarriage in August of 2009. Granted, I had shed many tears and for some time I felt animosity toward any pregnant woman I saw. I finally realized that I had missed having another child. However, I also realized that I wanted to be a parent to another child, and it didn't really matter anymore if this was my own biological child or not.

I believe the most insightful part of our training was meeting a couple who had adopted through LSS. They had waited two years to be placed with their son. When I saw that handsome little boy with the big brown eyes, I could tell he was the light of his parents' world.

It was then I knew we were doing the right thing. Yes, Ryan and I could no longer have a biological child, but I was looking forward to continuing with our adoption journey.

Chapter 80

The Picture Portfolio

I n September 2010, our home study was complete. The interview was painless even though I spent many hours cleaning the house. In retrospect, I believe the whole purpose of a home study is to see if your house is safe and child-friendly, not for the social worker to report on how clean it is!

After our home study, I worked many long hours on putting our portfolio together. This picture album tells your family story. I was so grateful for my brother's help. I am not computer savvy, but I have to say that the website and portfolio looked pretty darn impressive when it was finished.

I sent the portfolio off to the LSS office at the end of September 2010. Now I struggled with waiting for the phone to ring and for our social worker to tell us when a birth mother wanted a match meeting with us. I breathed deeply and kept telling myself that good things come to those who wait.

Chapter 81

Life's Lessons

I have to admit that along life's journey, I have learned a few things. I've learned I need to live each day to the fullest. Sometimes, it's easy to take those we love for granted, because we believe they will be around for a long, long time. But I'm here to tell you to enjoy each and every moment you have with your loved ones. You never know when they will be gone from your life.

Don't sweat the small stuff. This sounds like an overused phrase, but truly, life is too precious to worry about the littlest things.

All the struggles, grief, and heartbreak I have endured have made me the person I am today. Granted, I still have my quirks and faults, but these things have made me a stronger, healthier person. I can look back at my life and see that I've sometimes learned the hard way from my mistakes. It has taken me some time, but I have also learned to move forward and, as Don Pieper says, "create a new normal" for myself.

I'd like to end this story with a quote from Don Pieper. Don is a minister who was involved in a car accident that changed his life. The accident made him reflect on how we live our lives after a traumatic event. Don says, "If we're going to make the best of life, we have to get past the event that brought us pain and grow from it." I believe this is true, and I hope to continue to move forward in life with hope, love, and a sense of peacefulness. I know that God and my family are with me no matter what curveballs life may throw at me!